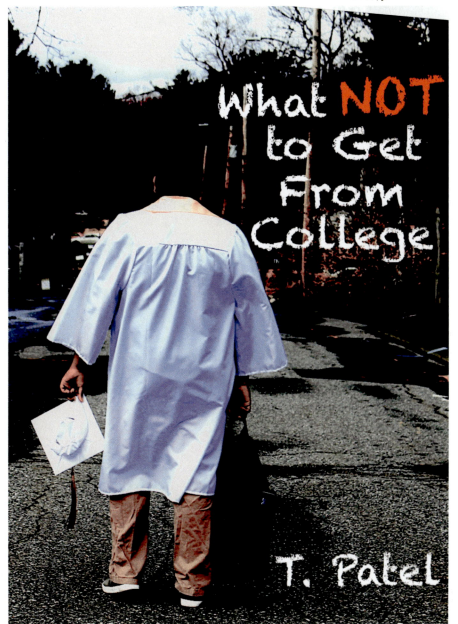

What NOT to Get from College

Written By: T. Patel

Published by Kindle Direct Publishing.

All rights are reserved. No part of this book may be reproduced in any manner without written permission of the author except in the cases of brief quotations for reviews.

Cover Design by T. Patel.

Contents

Acknowledgements — 2

Hyperlinks — 4

Introduction — 5

Chapter 1: Background in Science — 8

Chapter 2: Vaccine Preventable Diseases — 16

Chapter 3: Do I Have to Get the Flu Shot? — 37

Chapter 4: Meningitis — 43

Chapter 5: Let's Talk Sex. — 49

Chapter 6: How to Process Information — 61

Chapter 7: Myths — 77

Chapter 8: Autism — 81

Chapter 9: Ingredients — 92

Chapter 10: Create the Herd — 101

Conclusion — 106

References — 108

Acknowledgements

There are many people that I would like to acknowledge for the creation of this book. The first person has to be Dr. Cuchara. Without her Immunology and Vaccines classes, I wouldn't have even thought about writing a book. I relied heavily on the information from her classes as well as the sources that she provided.

I also wanted to acknowledge and thank all my peers from my BMS525 Vaccines course as their presentations, projects, and discussion helped me throughout the semester. The class presentations and discussions were very enlightening. I would have struggled to write a few of the chapters in this book if it weren't for these classmates.

Another "thank you" goes to my research group members. Although this book was written for my Vaccines course, my research from BMS482 played a large role in gaining information. Without our journal clubs, I certainly wouldn't have been able to write about more recent cases of diseases. I also would like to thank each of you for such an incredible research semester. It was so much more enjoyable because of our silly antics. (Dr. Cuchara, I promise we were working very hard when we weren't being silly).

I would also like to thank all the teachers and professors in my life that have helped me be where I am today. My first English professor really helped me learn who I was as a writer and without her, I wouldn't have had any confidence in writing this book. I also want to acknowledge my Honors Program director for addressing all my questions and worries throughout the semester.

I would also like to acknowledge all my friends and cousins. Your support is very much appreciated as I can be quite the handful when I am stressed out. It means so much to me that each of you listened to me talk about vaccines for the entire semester. It would have been very difficult for me to write this book if your encouragement and presence weren't there. (Also, thank you for reminding to eat food and take breaks while writing).

The next two people I have to acknowledge and thank are my siblings. Thank you for dealing with my last-minute book cover request. I know you didn't want to do it but it really meant a lot. Special shout outs to my brother for being the model for the cover and to my sister for taking the photo. Without them, the cover of this book would not be in existence. I appreciate it with all my heart.

Lastly, I would like to acknowledge my parents and grandmother. They had no idea I was writing this book. In fact, my grandmother has no way of reading it. However, these three people have done so much to bring me to the place that I am. Without their sacrifices and hard work, I wouldn't even have the opportunity to write this book.

I think I'm known for being too ambitious. When I first started this book, I had a very strong feeling I was going to give up. I was genuinely scared of failing myself. I tried keeping this project a secret but then realized that was a silly idea. Everyone who knew I was working on this throughout the semester was able to contribute to the creation of this book just by being there for me. Overall, thank you to everyone who supports me and all my overly ambitious goals. I don't think I'll stop being overly ambitious any time soon.

Hyperlinks

The original nature of this publication allowed for the usage of hyperlinks to various forms of online media such as videos and websites.

In order for paperback edition readers to receive the full experience, the following webpage has been created. The link below will have all the hyperlinks that were available in the original format of the book.

URL: https://goo.gl/FJMJaa

Thank you and enjoy reading!

Introduction

Welcome to College! If you're reading this book, you're probably about to start your first semester at your university or college! Or you've already started and wanted to know what this book was all about? Maybe you're just curious as to what one should not be getting at college? You could also be one of my many friends and family members who are slightly obligated to read this book for me? Regardless, you're going to learn about what someone shouldn't get from college. But first, let's think about what everyone wants from college.

As a freshly minted college student, new experiences and new beginnings are usually on the mind. There is a whole world of opportunity and you can finally start to explore it! I know that I really wanted to make new friends. I was excited to live in a new state. (Maybe you're going to school in a new country?) I was hopeful of finding new restaurants to love. I wanted to explore and travel to new places. I was also super excited to take my classes and learn information that'll actually matter to me.

I was excited for all the freedom. The freedom. Oh, the freedom. Being able to make your own decisions about what to eat, when to sleep, who to hang out with, everything. All these changes can be extremely exhilarating. However, they can also be super terrifying. What if I don't make new friends? What if I fail all my first exams? What if my professors think I'm stupid? What if they are all mean? What if I spend every Friday night in my room alone, eating ice cream and watching hours of Netflix? There are so many different concerns related to a college social life. (There is also nothing wrong with spending a Friday night watching Netflix and eating ice cream, it can be used as self-care, just to put that out there).

Making new friends. Taking major specific classes. Finding yourself as person. Developing new skills. Picking up new hobbies. Getting new ideas. Learning. A college degree and hopefully everything necessary to join the real world. Those are pretty typical things that someone expects to get from college, right?

During these years, there are going to be some serious learning curves. How does one study and manage time? How can you make sure you avoid serious weight gain (A.K.A. the feared Freshman 15!)? Maybe you don't know how to do laundry? Or maybe even more complicated things such as paying bills or keeping track of loans? Regardless, there are so many new skills and experiences that lie ahead.

Among all the excitement and fun, there's stress. A whole lot of stress. This stress may come from school work or relationships. They may be related to your family life back at home or they may be related to your health. There are so many different ways that stress will be brought into your life.

My goal for this book is to inform you of information that you most likely will not learn (unless you study the health sciences). This is all information that I wish I had learned before I went to college. It's an attempt of providing enough information for high school students or first year college students. For that reason, you'll notice that the book is fairly informal. In fact, I just wrote in first and second person multiple times which I know I learned is a big NO when writing formally. However, this book is supposed to try to replicate a conversation you could have with a friendly and knowledgeable upperclassman. After all, I am currently writing this as an upperclassman at my university. It is going to be a fairly one-sided conversation since it is a book but obviously you can talk to your friends, family members, peers and consult the internet if you have further questions.

So. The title of this book: What Not to Get from College?

What's that all about? (You know, aside from insane student debt what are you not supposed to get).

Let me ask you one question: Have you gotten your shots yet?

Shots? Like, basketball? Alcohol? Chances? The answer is no. I mean, vaccinations such as the flu shot. What does that have to do with college? Easy, you're about to go into the world. The world has many diseases. I mean, like so many. You're probably aware of many of them but don't know a lot of details.

I want to provide accurate knowledge regarding vaccines and vaccine preventable diseases. This information is very important for a few reasons. One reason is that for many young adults, our parents and medical professionals have made most of decisions up until this point. Many of you may never have questioned their decisions because why do we have to? Our parents make those decisions because they know best, right? However, maybe you should be making your decisions?

Another reason is that many people confuse opinion with fact. As you go through college, you're going to meet so many different people with so many different perspectives. You're going to find people who agree with you. You're going to find people who will not even listen to you. Knowing the difference and understanding the evidence are going to be pretty important when it comes to health care advice. There are people who try to sell their opinions as medical fact. That can be very dangerous.

Another reason is that before you go to your university, you're going to have to give them a copy of your immunization forms. For a good reason, your university is going to bring so many different people together from many different parts of the country and possibly the world. They need to make sure all your health records are in order and that you are healthy and protected. So, before you actually get to move into your dorm, make new friends and start new classes, you're probably going to have to go to the doctor to get cleared. This step is very simple but mundane. (It is super important!).

A final reason is that vaccines are very important and most people don't realize it. For that reason, I've written this book. Why? I'll be honest. I wrote this book as a project for my Vaccines course. The course required a "Change the World" project. For my project, I decided I wanted to write a book about vaccines in order to change the world for the better. I mostly wanted to share all the information that I learned from my

Immunology and my Vaccines courses. So, that is how we have arrived here. What Not to Get from College.

This book covers many topics related to medicine, scientific research, and health care. However, for actual all medical diagnoses, you should be going to an accredited health care professional. The purpose of this book is to be educational. Some of this information may be old news to you. Some of this may be very new. Some of it may confuse you. Some of it may make you very angry. All of this information will be right here in this book and you can refer to it whenever you need to. Now, I also want to point out that vaccines are a very controversial topic. You may be aware of this or you may not have been. Why are they controversial? If you keep reading you'll find out.

Chapter 1: Background in Science

How exactly do vaccines work? Are there tiny little wizards involved? Do we have tiny elves fighting off the diseases? Maybe tiny robots are injected into our bodies when we're born and that's how it all works. Those are all totally unrealistic explanations, but some would be totally cool. But in all seriousness, what is the science behind it all? Fair warning, this chapter is very science heavy (and I personally wish the mini wizards were involved).

This chapter is only going to give you a brief explanation of the immune system. If you find that you want to learn more about the specific nuances, I suggest doing more research or finding an anatomy and physiology textbook. You could also take an immunology course as that is a whole course devoted to just the immune system. I would highly suggest taking an immunology course in college if this is your field of interest.

Now, let's get started. You've probably heard of your immune system. It's the system in your body that protects you from getting sick. If you do get sick, it works extra hard to try to get you healthy again. Can you imagine living your life without a functioning immune system? You go grocery shopping with your mom and the next morning you have a fever. Or maybe you decide to go to the movies and someone sneezes and the next day you're sick in bed all day? For a person with a functioning immune system, it might be difficult to imagine what a world like that would be like. Yet, there are so many people living in the world with immune systems that aren't fully functioning or properly working!

What is the immune system? The immune system consists of a few organs that most people don't think about as being together. They include the skin, tonsils, thymus, bone marrow, spleen lymph nodes, bowels (intestines), and mucous membranes of the nose, throat, bladder and genitals[2]. The figure below shows each of these organs and their locations.

immune system organs

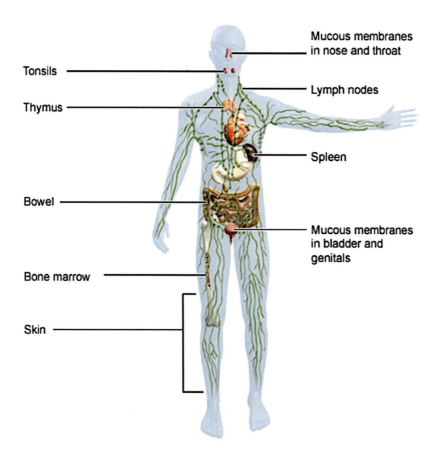

What are the parts of the immune system?

Figure 1. Diagram of the immune system [2]

The skin provides the first barrier to the outside world. If it's intact, it prevents many pathogens from entering. There are also chemicals and bacteria that reside on the skin that provide protection. The mucous membranes in your body have the same function. They stop pathogens from entering your body by capturing it in the mucous. stop enter- Meanwhile, the bone marrow and thymus are crucial in producing and developing the ance blood cells that essentially work the entire immune system. Your blood, specifically the white blood cells, are super important when it comes to monitoring the body. Some of the white blood cells are involved in recognizing and attacking the pathogens. The T-lymphocytes and B-lymphocytes (also known as T-cells and B-cells) are two important players. There are other white blood cells such as neutrophils, monocytes, eosinophils, and basophils that are also important in protecting the body.

The spleen's function depends on your age. For fetuses, the spleen actually produces the blood cells[2]. However, after birth, its main functions involve removing old red blood cells, storing and releasing different white blood cells, and storing and removing blood platelets. Other organs are also very important in how the system function. For instance, the lymph nodes work to create antibodies with the use of white blood cells and screen the blood. The tonsils and other tissues such as those in the bowels have white blood cells that monitor, detect and protect those parts of the body as well. The immune system is a few different organs that work together to provide protection. Its mechanisms can be very complex. However, it is also super cool because it remembers which foreign invaders attacked it. It, then, uses this memory to act quicker in recognizing and attacking the invaders the second time they attack[2].

Another important concept to understand involves the word "pathogen". Pathogens are microorganisms (typically, bacteria, fungi, and viruses) that can cause disease. This distinction is important because your body is covered with bacteria that do not harm you so they are not considered pathogenic. The human body is equipped with methods of determining which microorganisms are pathogenic and which are harmless. The immune system's main role is to recognize the pathogen and protect your body from harm.

How do these organs work together? There are two general ways the immune system works. There is the innate immune system and there is the adaptive immune system[3]. The adaptive immune system relies on recognition and is the main mechanism that is manipulated by vaccines. The innate immune system is nonspecific. The body doesn't recognize specific pathogens. Instead, this system notices that there is a foreign invader and it uses a few different ways to attack the problem[3]. Essentially, the body can tell something is wrong, but isn't sure of what specifically is happening. Since it doesn't know what's happening it doesn't create a specific plan. Instead, it has broader methods of killing off the pathogens.

There are a few different players to how the body can kill off the pathogen nonspecifically. These players are cells known as phagocytes, macrophages, and natural killer cells[3]. There are other white cells such as neutrophils, eosinophils, basophils and monocytes that are very important players in the innate immune system[3]. These cells work together while your body feels "sick". Typically, during a fever, these are the cells that work to get you healthy again. The fever raises the temperature so your cells can work faster to repair any damage and get you back on your feet. The body also goes into inflammation. Imagine getting cut, after some time, the cut feels very warm and starts to swell a little bit. This process happens because your body recognized that you got hurt. It directs more blood to that area so that repairs can occur. These are only a few ways the innate immune system works. After all, it nonspecifically protects the body by keeping all pathogens out or killing them off with chemicals. For instance, the skin is actually part of the innate immune system because of those properties[3].

However, as mentioned, the body is also capable of producing specific responses to very specific invaders. This type of system is known as the adaptive immune system.

How does the recognition really work? There are cells that recognize antigens and distinguishes them between self and non-self[3]. Except, what's an antigen? Antigens are proteins. The ones that we are specifically talking about elicit an immune response. The proteins can be detached parts of a virus or bacteria[3]. They can also still be attached to the entire bacterium or virus. The antigen is basically a little marker that the body recognizes as foreign[3]. It can tell that it is not you. Since it is not you, it can attack it.

Proteins

The T cells and the B cells are the main players for the adaptive immune system. The pathways of how they work are very complex and complicated. In fact, the adaptive immune system can be further divided. However, the main concept of how the adaptive immune system is really all a person needs to know in order to understand vaccines.

The adaptive immune system relies on the T-cells and B-cells to recognize the pathogens in the body. These T-cells are capable of destroying all the pathogens or pathogen infected cells in the body. The B-cells recognize and create antibodies. These antibodies are proteins that can attach to the antigens of the pathogens. These antibodies have a few functions. The antibodies don't do the direct killing but they work with other white blood cells. The B-cells are also capable of multiplying and producing lots of antibodies. The B-cells can also create memory cells which just hang around the body until the pathogen enters the body again[3]. Overall, the adaptive immune system is important for recognizing specific pathogens and creating antibodies. This process is exactly what vaccinations use to work.

memory

The immune system can also be divided into two types of immunities. There is passive immunity and there is active immunity. What's the difference? Passive immunity is basically getting immunity without ever encountering the disease-causing agent. In other words, another animal or person's already made antibodies are placed within a person so they do not have to produce those antibodies. The person is "passively" getting protection.

Where does this passive immunity come from? There are a few ways. The first method was there when you were first born. After emerging from the womb, a baby still relies on their mother for protection. Whatever your mom is immune to, you are likely to have received her antibodies. She gives you this type of immunity in the womb. Once out of the womb, a mother can breastfeed her child and continue giving them passive immunity. This phenomenon occurs because there are antibodies that are in the breastmilk. (It's part of why some people strongly advocate for breastmilk instead of formula, however, that is an entirely different topic). As you can see, passive immunity can be pretty great. However, it is a temporary form of immunity. According to the CDC pink book, after birth, full-term babies have antibodies from their mother for about two months. The antibodies from the mother last for up to a year. Essentially, for the first few months of life, babies have the same antibodies as their mothers[1]. They rely on this protection as their immune system finishes development.

need AB from mom while system is still developing

There are also other forms of passive immunity. Passive immunity can also come from receiving blood transfusions or other blood products. There are also other forms of antibodies that are used in modern medicine. These forms are homologous pooled human antibody, homologous human hyperimmune globulin, and heterologous hyperimmune serum. The homologous pooled human antibody is basically a combination of a specific antibody (IgG) from various adult, human donors in the United States. These antibodies have a lot of variability as they come from so many different people. They are often used to treat people after exposure to hepatitis A, measles, and for some congenital immunodeficiencies. The second form, homologous human hyperimmune globulin, are products made from donated human blood plasma. This form contains high amounts of antibodies made for very specific diseases. These products are given to people who have been exposed to hepatitis B, rabies, tetanus, and varicella[1].

The final product, heterologous hyperimmune serum is known as an antitoxin. These antitoxins are typically produced in animals, specifically horses. This product only contains antibodies against one antigen. In the United States, this antitoxin is used to treat people who have been infected with botulism and diphtheria. This product does have one disadvantage as it causes some people to get sick. They get sick from an immune reaction to the proteins from the horses that were used to produce the antitoxins. Clearly, there are a few methods of receiving passive immunity. However, most of them are used after the person is infected or as a post-exposure prophylaxis[1]. Again, this form of passive immunity is very important and useful, however, it is temporary.

The other type of immunity is known as active immunity. Active immunity is when a person comes into direct contact with the antigen. This type of immunity lasts longer than passive immunity. It is often referred to as "natural" immunity[3]. As mentioned, vaccines work by utilizing this type of immunity. In active immunity, the antigen comes into contact with specific immune cells. The immune cells respond and talk to each and create antibodies. The antibodies are released into the rest of the blood and basically bind to the pathogen and act as a marker for the immune cells[3]. The antibodies also float around in the blood and last a while. When the body encounters this same pathogen again, there is a faster response because the antibodies and memory cells already exist.

Table 1. Comparison of Passive and Active Immunities[1]

Passive Immunity	Active Immunity
Temporary	Lasts for many years; Potentially Life-Long
From Other Animals/People	Your Own Body

Vaccines focus on creating a memory response so that there is a quicker recognition and attack. The vaccines contain the antigens. These antigens are unable to give the disease to the recipient. The antigens do not elicit the symptoms of that disease. For example, when you get the chickenpox vaccine (varicella), you do not experience the itchy chickenpox rash. In terms of immune responses, they can be generally categorized as primary and secondary responses. The primary response occurs the very first time the body encounters the pathogen. It takes some time, a few days to maybe a week, for the body to create this response. As mentioned, the adaptive immune system can remember when certain pathogens attack. The secondary response occurs any time after the first exposure. Since all the cells are at the ready, the response is much quicker and lasts a shorter amount of time. The secondary response can occur as many times as the person is exposed to the pathogen[3].

Vaccines act as the first exposure to the pathogen. They basically help the body experience the primary immune response earlier so that way any exposure to the actual pathogen elicits a secondary immune response. For that reason, it typically takes some time (example: two weeks) for the vaccines to create an immune response in humans and provide actual protection. Time is the key.

As there are many different pathogens in the world, there are a few different types of vaccines. Overall, there are two main categories of vaccines. The first category are live attenuated vaccines. "Attenuated" means weakened. The second category is inactivated vaccines. Within the inactivated vaccines, there are further subdivisions known as killed, toxoid, recombinant/subunit, and conjugate. Each type of vaccine is prepared differently and have their own advantages and disadvantages. The vaccines also have their own methods of being prepared.

For instance, live-attenuated vaccines are produced by taking the virus or bacteria and growing it many (I mean, MANY) times in non-human cells. The pathogen is still alive and capable of replicating. It needs to replicate in the cells in order for the antibodies to be produced. However, since it is still alive this type of vaccine is not given to immunocompromised populations because there is always a chance of mutation[1]. Immunocompromised populations include pregnant women, very young children/babies, geriatric people (the elderly), cancer patients, people with autoimmune disorders, and transplant patients. You probably know someone who is immunocompromised and don't even realize it!

The concern is that the weakened pathogen reverts back to being infectious to humans. A healthy human could handle that reversion whereas an immunocompromised person is more at risk of dying. This type of vaccine is capable of giving lifelong immunity, however, titers are always recommended in order to ensure the antibody counts are high enough. A titer, by the way, is a measurement of how many antibodies for a specific disease can be detected in your blood. In order to obtain a titer, a health care professional has to draw some blood (yes, another needle).

Moving on, the killed vaccines are basically what they sound like. The pathogen is killed physically through the use of light, heat or chemicals[1]. Regardless, the pathogen is killed so that it can no longer hurt people. There is no way for it to replicate and there is no way for it mutate. It's dead. These vaccinations are great because they can be given to anyone. However, they require booster shots as they cannot give lifelong immunity[1].

Toxoid vaccines are pretty interesting because they don't require the whole microorganism. The pathogens for these vaccines excrete toxins. These toxins are isolated and inactivated so that they can no longer hurt humans. These vaccines are useful because it doesn't require the pathogen and can be given to immunocompromised populations. The next type of vaccine is sometimes referred to as subunit or recombinant. Personally, in my immunology course, I used those interchangeably. Over time, scientists may come to a consensus as to what it should be called or maybe one name will just phase out. Anyway, the recombinant vaccine is produced by genetic engineering. Don't get angry or scared about that just yet! Essentially, specific genes are isolated from the pathogens and can be inserted into another cell such as yeast cells. The yeast cells can replicate and produce the protein that the gene codes. This protein can be produced and isolated. These proteins are pure and are used in the vaccines as the antigens[1].

The final type of vaccine is known as conjugate vaccines. These vaccines are for specific bacteria. Why bacteria? Bacteria have a sugar component known as a polysaccharide. These sugars make creating vaccines for young children a little difficult. For that reason, these sugars undergo a process known as "conjugation". This process is basically taking sugar and adding it to a protein so that different cells attack the protein and create an effective immune response. These vaccines also need booster shots as they do not provide lifelong immunity[1].

Those are the different types of vaccines and just a few advantages and disadvantages that are associated with these vaccines. Another important note is that these vaccines do require specific storage. Some of them need to be maintained at very specific temperatures and they have to be stored in specific manners as well. These specific storage requirements can be a disadvantage depending on the situation.

Table 2. Examples of Types of Vaccines and their Diseases[1]

Type of Vaccine	Live Attenuated	Killed	Toxoid	Recombinant/ Subunit	Conjugate
Diseases	Measles	Influenza	Diphtheria	Hepatitis B	Hemophilius influenza
	Mumps	Polio	Tetanus	Human Papillomavirus	Meningococcal
	Rotavirus	Hepatitis A		Pertussis	Pneumococcal
	Rubella				
	Varicella				

Those are some of the types of vaccines that exist in the world today. There are many more that exist for other diseases. There are also many vaccines that are currently under research. For instance, when the Ebola outbreak occurred sometime around 2015, there was a large amount of pressure for scientists to create a vaccine for it. The same happened with the Zika virus outbreaks that occurred around the end of 2016. There are so many different parts to the immune system and so many different pathogens. It's a wonder how scientists are even capable of figuring all of this out.

Think about it, these are tiny little organisms that you can't see. On these organisms, there are little proteins that need to be discovered or figured out. Once that information is obtained, scientists have to figure how to make a vaccine that is safe enough to use in humans. All of this work clearly requires large amounts of research over long periods of times with so many different scientists. Except, there's one very crucial question.

Do vaccines even work? As my high school French teacher always used to say "The proof is in the pudding!" Yes, vaccines do work! There is ample evidence to show that the prevalence of disease has decreased over the years. What does that even mean? How can you be sure? Keep reading and you'll find out!

Chapter 2: Vaccine Preventable Diseases

At this point in your life, you've probably received many vaccines. The vaccine recommendations for the United States are determined by the Centers for Disease Control and Prevention (they're also known as the CDC to make everyone's lives easier). Their recommendations are based off of scientific evidence and consultations.

Some of the vaccines that are recommended include: MMR, rotavirus, varicella, polio, and tetanus. These names and abbreviations may sound familiar to you. If not, that's perfectly fine! You're probably going to recognize some of them when you complete your vaccination forms for your college/university.

Let's discuss diseases. There are many diseases that we can't really figure out so they don't have solutions or cures. Some diseases are non-communicable (meaning they cannot be spread from person to person). Some examples of non-communicable diseases include: obesity, hypertension, and diabetes. Some diseases are communicable (meaning they are infectious and can be spread from person to person) such as the flu, chickenpox, and measles.

I'm going to focus on communicable diseases. Many of the communicable diseases that used to plague much of the human population have vaccines. They are known as "vaccine preventable diseases" (or VPDs for short). For that reason, many people don't even know about the devastating consequences of these diseases that can occur. In a way, countries like the United States, almost take it for granted that the prevalence for these diseases have dropped significantly.

Measles

We live in a time where we are very lucky that most children do not get measles. However, the disease still exists and there are people who refuse getting vaccinated against it. For that reason, there are still sporadic measles cases that pop up. For instance, you may have heard of the measles cases that were linked to Disneyland in 2015?

In 2015, a measles outbreak began in Disneyland. There were around 59 cases of measles. From those cases, 42 cases were linked to Disneyland. There were 34 patients who were from California. Of those 34, 28 patients were not vaccinated against the disease. Of the 28 patients that were not vaccinated, six of the patients were babies who were unable to get vaccinated as they were too young. Out of the 34 patients, five were fully vaccinated but still contracted the disease and one was partially vaccinated[5]. How could that have happened? Simple, there are at least two ways that measles becomes an issue in the United States. The first way is someone who is unvaccinated travels to another country and brings it back. The second way is if someone from another country visits and they have the disease. As time continues to move by, other sporadic cases and outbreaks of measles occur. Except, what is this disease?

Measles is caused by a virus. The virus is spread through a respiratory transmission which means that it spreads through coughing, sneezing, close personal or direct contact with someone who is already infected. A person can infect those around them four days before the rash shows up and up to four days after the rash occurs. The virus remains active in the air or on surfaces up to two hours after being spread (basically, it is still contagious for two hours after someone coughs or sneezes)[2].

The first sign of the disease is usually a high fever that starts 10 to 12 days after exposure to the virus. The fever can last from four to seven days. Other signs and symptoms include a runny nose, a cough, conjunctivitis (the red and watery eyes), and white spots on the cheeks. Measles is specifically characterized by a rash that starts from the hairline and moves its way to the face and upper neck. The rash spreads throughout the body until it reaches the hands and feet. The tell-tale sign of measles is the occurrence of Koplik spots the in mucous membranes. Basically, spots that are blue/white show up specifically in the mouth[2].

There are also many complications from measles. Death is often times caused by the complications. These complications are most common among children under the age of five and adults over the age of 30. Complications include blindness, encephalitis (that's an infection caused by swelling of the brain), severe diarrhea and dehydration, ear infections, and respiratory infections such as pneumonia[2]. Historically, measles was known to affect basically all children under the age of five years old[1]. The bar graph in figure 1 shows that children under five and over the age of 20 were typically hospitalized the most and experienced pneumonia[1]. This graph shows how these two age groups experienced more complications than those in between the ages of five and 20.

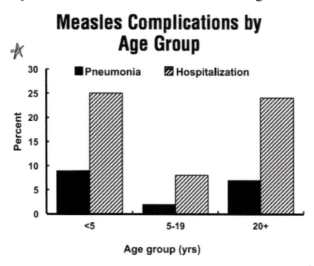

Figure 1. Complications of measles by age group[1]

According to the WHO, before the measles vaccination, there would be measles epidemics every two to three years and caused approximately 2.6 million deaths each year. The graph from the CDC, in figure 2, shows how there has been a decrease in the cases of measles since the introduction of the vaccine. However, the graph below it also shows how there was a resurgence of measles in the United States around 1989[1]. Also, note how these are statistics for the United States. According to the WHO, measles is still an issue in many developing countries such as in Africa and Asia. There is no treatment for the virus[1]. The disease only occurs in humans and can only be spread by humans[1]. Since there is no treatment, prevention is the best way to avoid such epidemics.

Measles is not safer for someone to naturally contract measles. If a healthy person gets measles, their bodies will be immunosuppressed for two to three years after they get the disease. Imagine living three years without a healthy immune system! Why does this happen? Once a person has measles, their bodies have a difficult time developing the B-cells and T-cells[6]. Think about this complication further. Children who are typically five years old contract this disease. After they contract this disease, they are immunocompromised and still at risk for many other diseases such as the other childhood VPDs.

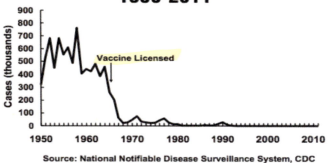

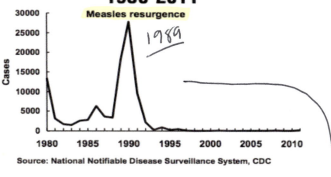

Measles Resurgence—United States, 1989-1991

- Cases
  - 55,622
- Age group affected
  - children younger than five years
- Deaths
  - 123

Figure 2. CDC graphs showing the cases of measles from 1950 to 2011 and resurgence of measles from 1980 to 2011[1]

Mumps

Mumps is another disease that many people are very lucky not to experience. What are mumps? Mumps is also a childhood disease that is caused by a virus. It is caused by a similar type of virus as the measles virus. It incubates in the body for 12 to 25 days. Within this time period, it can spread to various places in the body including meninges (tissues that protect your brain), salivary glands, the pancreas, the testes and the ovaries[1].

The signs and symptoms of the disease are myalgia (fancy word for pain in muscles), anorexia, malaise (another fancy word for discomfort or uneasiness), headache, and a low-grade fever. The complications of mumps include many words that end with "itis." This ending means "inflammation." The many complications of mumps include: orchitis, pancreatitis, parotitis, meningitis, and appendicitis. Orchitis is a common in young men who have past puberty and it is the inflammation in the testes. Men who experience orchitis are at risk for sterility. Pancreatitis is the inflammation of the pancreas. Parotitis is the inflammation of the parotid gland (the parotid is a salivary gland that can be found in your mouth and helps with digestion). Meningitis is the inflammation of the meninges which are an important tissue that protect your brain. There is also appendicitis which is the inflammation of the appendix. There is also oophoritis which is the inflammation of the ovaries but that is not as likely to happen as the other inflammations. Another complication of mumps is deafness. Some people experienced deafness in one ear or both ears[1].

Parotitis is the most common symptom of mumps. It can be unilateral or bilateral which means it can happen on one side to one gland or to both glands. It usually occurs within the first two days and can cause an earache and tenderness on the jaw. The inflammation can take a week and up to seven days to go away[1].

Mumps is also a human disease that is spread through respiratory transmissions. Similar to measles, mumps can be spread through the air by coughing or sneezing. It can also be spread through direct contact with saliva. Mumps differs from measles in that some people remain asymptomatic (they don't have symptoms) but are still capable of spreading the disease[1].

For instance, the graph in figure 3 shows how the vaccine helped decrease the number of mumps cases significantly.

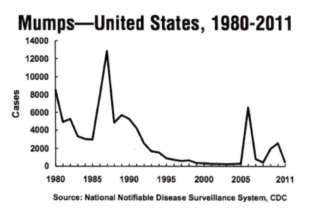

Figure 3. CDC graph showing cases of mumps from 1980 to 2011[1]

The figure above shows trends in mumps cases in the United States between 1980 and 2011. The graph shows how there have been fluctuations in cases between these two years. As you can see, there is an overall decline in the number of cases. As the vaccination rates fluctuate, there have been cases of mumps in places such as college campus. According to a study performed at Harvard, there have been more mumps outbreaks on college campuses as of 2006[3]. This example is one reason why college students should care about their immunization statuses. What if the mumps end up on your college campus? Are you immune enough to avoid getting sick?

Rubella

What is rubella? Rubella is also another childhood disease. However, it is very dangerous for pregnant women to contract. This disease is also caused by a virus and has respiratory transmission. The virus can take up to five to seven days to spread throughout a person's blood after exposure. Similar to measles and mumps, rubella also has a rash but it is not as prominent. In older children and adults, rubella has a low-grade fever, malaise, lymphadenopathy, and other upper respiratory symptoms along with the rash. The rash occurs 14 to 17 days after exposure. In adults, there may also be arthralgia and arthritis[1].

As mentioned, this disease is a major concern for pregnant women. The virus can infect a fetus during pregnancy because it can pass through the placenta. This disease is known as Congenital Rubella Syndrome or CRS. When a fetus is infected with the virus, the infection can affect all the organs of its body. CRS can lead to fetal death or a premature birth. If the baby survives, deafness is the most common issue after birth. However, there can also be eye defects such as cataracts, glaucoma, retinopathy, and microphthalmia. There are also cardiac defects such as patent ductus, arteriosus, ventricular septal defect, pulmonic stenosis, and coarctation of the aorta. There are also neurological abnormalities such as microcephaly, and mental retardation. Among the other issues that can occur there are bone lesions, splenomegaly, hepatitis, and thrombocytopenia with purpura. If you are curious, below is a table that explains what all of those means. However, the bottom line is if a pregnant woman is infected, the baby can have some serious problems. There is also a higher risk for babies of developing diabetes or autism if they develop CRS[1].

Table 2. Complications and Birth Defects from Rubella[1]

Type of Defect	Complications	Definitions/Explanations
Eye Defects	Cataracts	Lead to blurred vision
	Glaucoma	Increased pressure in eye
	Retinopathy	Diseased retina
	Microphthalmia	Abnormally small eyeballs
Cardiac Defects	Patent Ductus Arteriosus	Failure of blood vessels in fetal heart
	Ventricular Septal Defect	Hole in the ventricles of the heart
	Pulmonic Stenosis	Blood flow from the heart to pulmonary artery stops (arteries connecting the lungs)
	Coarctation of the Aorta	Aorta narrows (connects heart to rest of body)
Neurological Defects	Microencephaly	Smaller head
	Intellectual Disabilities	Slower or abnormal brain development that impedes some function
Other Defects that were listed…	Bone Lesions	Destruction of bones
	Splenomegaly	Abnormally large spleen
	Hepatitis	Liver inflammation
	Thrombocytopenia with Purpura	Disorder that leads to bleeding and bruising

You're probably thinking, why is this disease something I should care about? First of all, this could have been you when you were chilling out in your mom's womb. If she were not vaccinated, there could have been a chance you could have been born with these issues. You're probably reading this and thinking "luckily that didn't happen" but it could have.

Imagine an elementary school. There are some children who are vaccinated and some children who are not vaccinated. This school has many hardworking teachers who just want to make a difference in the lives of their students. There is one teacher and she is incredibly happy because she just found out she was pregnant! One day, she goes to school and she notices one of her students isn't feeling very well. She takes that student aside and sends her to the nurse. Later that week, it turns out this student was not vaccinated against rubella. This student was contagious and capable of spreading it to her classmates and to her teacher. Had the teacher not been vaccinated, her baby was at risk. What about mothers who were not vaccinated as children though?

An important part of the MMR (measles, mumps, and rubella vaccine) is that it cannot be given to certain immunocompromised individuals. Pregnant women cannot get vaccinated until after pregnancy[1]. Babies are not able to get the vaccine until they are 12 months old[1]. That's a whole year without protection! The vaccine also cannot be given to older adults, transplant patients, or cancer patients undergoing chemotherapy. Basically, any person whose immune system is not properly functioning cannot receive the vaccine.

Polio

Once upon a time, poliomyelitis (polio for short) really scared people. There were children dying every single summer. It was normal for children to go away one summer and come autumn, their best friends may have gotten polio. Again, we're lucky to rarely see polio. Just for a second, imagine going back to second grade to find out your best friend died.

What exactly is polio? The most well-known complication of polio is paralysis. However, the paralysis is actually not as prevalent as many people think[1].

Polio is caused by a virus. It is spread through a fecal-oral route and it can also be spread through an oral-oral route. How can so many people be infected by a fecal-orally transmitted disease? Contaminated food and water are the main culprits. The virus enters through the mouth and enters the gastrointestinal tract. From there it replicates and can be shed through the feces. The virus makes its way to the bloodstream and can make its way to the central nervous system. Once it is in the central nervous system, the known symptoms of polio can manifest[1].

The initial symptoms of polio are fever, fatigue, headache, vomiting, stiffness of the neck, and pain in the limbs[2]. There are two types of polio that a person can experience. There is the non-paralytic polio and the paralytic polio. The non-paralytic polio has an incubation period of three to six days while the paralytic polio has an incubation period of 7 to 21 days[1].

According to the CDC, 72% of all polio infections in children were asymptomatic[1]. These children carried polio but did not experience any of the symptoms. They were still able to spread it to other people[1]. In terms of the paralytic cases, there were three categories that the cases could have been characterized. These categories are spinal polio, bulbar polio and a combination of spinal and bulbar polio.

The worst-case scenarios for polio were paralysis of the lungs. In these cases, children were placed in machines known as "iron lungs" which mechanically helped them breathe. Some children also experienced paralysis to the point where there was no recovery.

There are three known strains of the virus that causes polio (P1, P2 and P3)[1]. Contracting one strain of polio does not mean that the person is immune to the other two strains of polio. In fact, the person would have to contract all three strains in order to be immune.

There is no cure for polio. Once a person contracts the disease, they have it. The only way to protect people is from prevention. Polio is also a disease the only infects humans. There are no animal carriers or reservoirs. As of 1999, strain 2 of the wildtype polio virus has been completely eradicated[7].

The figure below shows the number of polio cases that the United States experienced between the 1950s and 2010. In figure 4, the graph shows how the introduction of the inactivated vaccine was able to decrease the number of cases substantially. Then there was a slight increase around the 1960s and another decrease shortly after.

The maps in figures 5 and 6 show the prevalence of polio in 1988 and 2012[1]. The first map shows the world with many cases of polio that still need to be eliminated[1]. The second map shows what happened after years of vaccination campaigns[1]. These two maps show a stark difference in the prevalence of the wildtype polio cases.

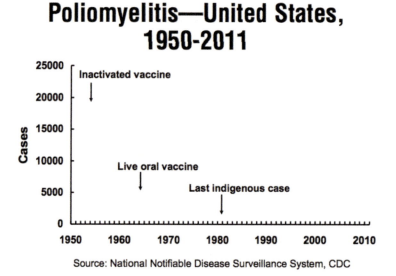

Figure 4. CDC graph that shows the trends of polio cases in United States[1]

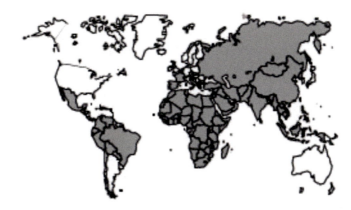

Figure 5. Prevalence of polio in 1988[1]

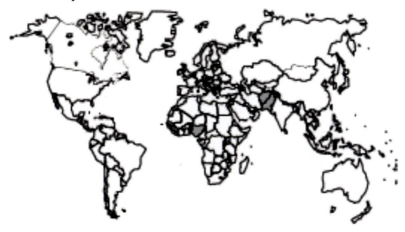

Figure 6. World map showing places where polio is still prevalent in 2012 [1]

Rotavirus

I'll be honest, before I even took my immunology course, I don't think I've ever heard of rotavirus. What's rotavirus? Rotavirus is similar to polio in that it is transmitted through the oral-fecal route. Again, what that means is that fecal matter that enters through the mouth can have this virus and infects people. In places without or very few sanitation programs, contaminated water and food is often an issue. This issue is seen in many developing countries. That does not mean that it only happens in developing countries. Even in developed countries, such as the United States, there are many people who do not wash their hands properly. You're probably cringing but yes, there are many people who do not wash their hands well enough. In fact, my freshman year of college, I witnessed many girls walk out of the bathroom without washing their hands at all. I still see that happen. (Yes, super gross!)

Rotavirus can remain in the environment for weeks or months after exposure if there has not been any method of disinfection. Since it can remain the environment, fomites are a concern. Fomites are basically objects that can help the virus stay alive. Clothing, water bottles, food, and so many other items can hold a virus or bacteria and you may not even know it[1].

Rotavirus does exist in some other mammals *but cannot transfer to humans*; however, those strains are very distinct from the type that infects humans. It is extremely rare that an animal rotavirus will infect a human. For that reason, t is still considered a human disease[1].

The first infection of rotavirus does not lead to an immunity to the disease. According to the CDC, only 38% of children who had contracted rotavirus have protection against the disease. However, there is an increased immunity each time a person contracts the disease. However, the symptoms of this disease may make you think twice about naturally getting infected.

The symptoms of rotavirus are diarrhea and fevers. The diarrhea can occur within 48 hours of being infected. Since this disease predominantly affects children in developing countries, there is a risk for severe diarrhea (as opposed to just diarrhea), dehydration, electrolyte imbalances, and metabolic acidosis. Children who are immunocompromised may experience some gastroenteritis and have abnormalities in organs such as the liver and kidneys[1].

Why should we care about rotavirus? It seems like there are other diseases to be worried about. The vaccine has definitely helped decrease numbers. According to the CDC, before the vaccine was available, there was an estimated 3 million cases per year. For the most part, children were infected before the age of 5 years old. There were about 20 to 60 deaths due to the virus[1].

Diphtheria

Diphtheria is another childhood disease that many of us are very lucky to have never experienced. It is a little different from the other diseases that I have mentioned already. Instead of being caused by a virus, diphtheria is caused by a bacterium. It is caused by *Corynebacterium diphtheriae* which explains why the disease is called "diphtheria". Naturally, the human body has different types of *Corynebacterium* that like to hang out on the skin or in the nose[1].

However, *C. diphtheriae* is different because it produces a toxin that can harm people. The toxin stops proteins from being built. Proteins are essential for the structure and function of the cells. The toxin can also cause major issues such as myocarditis and neuritis. Myocarditis is the inflammation of a layer of tissue in the heart while neuritis is the inflammation of the optic nerve in the eye. There may also be issues such as a low blood platelet count which is known as thrombocytopenia or proteins may leak into urine which is known as proteinuria[1].

The symptoms of diphtheria depend on the location that is infected. A person can experience anterior nasal diphtheria, pharyngeal and tonsillar diphtheria, laryngeal diphtheria and cutaneous diphtheria. In anterior nasal diphtheria, the symptoms feel very similar to the common cold. It progresses to include a discharge from the nose that includes pus and mucus. This discharge can have a tinge of blood as well. The disease can be treated if it is addressed quickly.

The pharyngeal and tonsillar diphtheria (throat and tonsils) are the most common sites of infection. When the pharynx is infected, a person will feel malaise, a sore throat, anorexia, and a low-grade fever around 101° F. A bluish-white membrane will form and extend around the tonsils and soft palate of the throat after two to three days. This membrane can change to green or black if there is bleeding. If the infection is extensive, there is a possibility that the person may not be able to breathe due to a blockage created by the membrane[1].

Some patients are capable of recovering from this infection without treatment. If a person does not receive treatment, there is a chance that the person will develop prostration which is lying down and not moving). The patient's skin may lose its color. The patient could develop a rapid pulse or lose mental function and consciousness. The patient could go into a coma. The person is at risk of dying within the six to ten-day mark of the infection[1].

For the laryngeal diphtheria, the symptoms include a fever, hoarseness, and a barking cough. In this infection, there is a chance that there is an airway obstruction (fancy words for airway being blocked). A person is at risk for developing a coma or death[1].

According to the CDC, cutaneous diphtheria (homeless people) is mostly associated with people who are homeless. In this form of infection, there is a rash or there can be ulcers. There can also be infections of the mucous membranes such as conjunctiva or in the vaginal area and sometimes in the external ear canal[1].

Complications for diphtheria, as mentioned, include death, myocarditis, and neuritis. The myocarditis may occur earlier during the infection. It could occur much later and cause heart failure as well. The neuritis usually affects motor nerves but can completely resolve itself. Often times, there is paralysis of the soft palate. There may even be paralysis of eye muscles, limbs, and diaphragm (which is pretty scary considering that organ controls your breathing). Some other complications include otitis media and respiratory insufficiency. Otitis media is an infection of the eardrum[1]. — eardrum infection

The treatment for this includes antitoxin and antibiotics. The antitoxin will be more effective in some areas than in other areas. An interesting fact about the antitoxin is that it was developed from horses. (Part of the reason why animal research is super important except it should be done ethically!) The antitoxin is able to neutralize (or undo the effects of) the free-floating toxin[1].

When the bacteria infect humans, the toxins are released into the cells and tissues. If the toxin is already stuck inside the tissues, the antitoxin can't go in and get rid of the toxin. The antitoxin can only help prevent the toxin from spreading and the disease from progressing further. The patient is also given antibiotics. These antibiotics are usually erythromycin or penicillin G. They are given either orally or by injection. Once a person is on the antibiotics after 48 hours, they are not contagious

As mentioned, an antitoxin is used to prevent the toxin from spreading throughout the body. This antitoxin cannot be used a preventative measure[1]. For that reason, scientists researched and created a vaccine.

Humans are a reservoir for *C. diphtheriae* and they are usually asymptomatic. During outbreaks, children are often carriers of this bacteria. The bacteria's transmission is respiratory. It can also be spread through contact with the skin and sometimes, but very rarely, through fomites[1].

In the figures below, there are graphs that show the cases of diphtheria in the United States. The graph in figure 7 shows that cases from 1940 to 2011. The graph shows a major drop in cases around 1950 and then stays closer to zero cases until 2011. In comparison, the graph in figure 8 shows there were fluctuations in cases between 1980 and 2011[1]. These two graphs show very similar information. The important difference is the scale used to show the amount of cases. The first graph had a larger scale with more cases while the second graph had a smaller scale with fewer graphs. Similar data is shown but the presentation differs. This difference is very important in understanding scientific studies as the graphs can show very different stories. The first graph shows that everything is going well, at least, generally speaking. The second graph shows more details and provides a clearer depiction. Remember that data presentation is important when reading scientific studies.

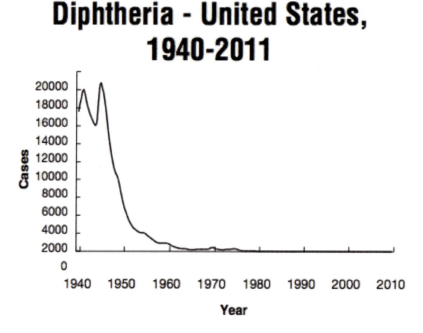

Figure 7. Cases of diphtheria from 1940 to 2011 according to the CDC[1]

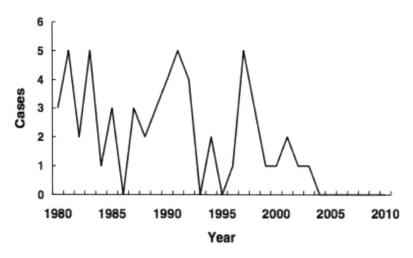

Figure 8. Cases of diphtheria from 1980 to 2011 according to the CDC[1]

Pertussis

You have probably heard of "whooping cough." The scientific word for it is "pertussis." Pertussis is also caused by a bacterium. This bacterium is *Bordetella pertussis.* This bacterium is similar to diphtheria in that it also has a toxin. The *B. pertussis* bacteria is a little creepy because of how it infects your body. It enters through the respiratory tract through droplets and secretions. Once inside the lungs, the bacteria attach to the cilia (these are tiny little projections on the inside of your lungs). After they attach to the cilia, the bacteria release the toxin which then paralyzes the cilia. The overall result is inflammation of the respiratory tract[1].

The clinical infection of this disease can be divided into three stages. The first stage involves a very runny nose, sneezing, a low-grade fever, and a cough similar to a cough from the common cold. However, the cough slowly becomes more severe over a course of one to two weeks[1].

The stage is usually when pertussis is actually noticed. This stage is when a person has bursts of rapid coughs that causes difficulty with breathing. The person has a difficult time clearing the mucus in their lungs (which is typically the reason for the cough). These attacks are characterized by the "whooping cough" sound. After a whooping cough episode, the person may look blue (the scientific description is "cyanotic"). The person may even vomit afterwards and be very tired. The final stage is a very gradual recovery. The cough disappears after two to three weeks[3]. However, the person may experience whooping cough attacks for months after the pertussis[1].

The main complications of this disease include death as well as pneumonia. There are chances of neurological complications such as seizures and encephalopathy. The neurological complications are more likely to occur in infants. Some other complications include otitis media, anorexia, and dehydration[1].

There may be complications that occur from pressure effects such as pneumothorax (collapsed lung), epistaxis (nose bleed), subdural hematomas (pooling of blood between brain and brain tissue), hernias (displacement of organ such as intestines), and rectal prolapse (the large intestine slips out the anus). Some complications that can happen to adolescents and adults include difficulty sleeping (probably due to all the coughing), urinary incontinence (no bladder control), pneumonia, and rib fractures[1].

The treatment for pertussis involves antibiotics. The antibiotics that are usually given are azithromycin, clarithromycin, and erythromycin. The antibiotics kills the bacteria from the secretions. Early treatment is very important. The treatment may also be given to people who live in close quarters with the infected person for obvious reasons that these people are at risk for contracting the bacteria themselves[1].

Much like all the other disease, this disease is also a human disease[1]. That means people give it to each other and animals are not often seen. Even though there are lower numbers in the United States, pertussis still exists very commonly in the rest of the world. According to the WHO, in 2016, there were 139,535 reported cases of pertussis and 89,000 estimated deaths due to pertussis[8].

This graph in figure 9 shows the trend in pertussis cases in the United States over time. Notice how over time, there are decreases and increases between the years of 1940 and around 1965. Then notice how there is a decrease and then almost a flat line between 1970 to 2000. Sadly, notice how there is an increase in cases after 2000 and around 2010. What could have happened around that time period that caused the number of cases to rise?

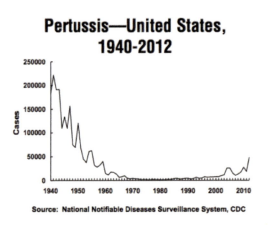

Figure 9. Cases of pertussis in the United States between 1940 to 2012 from the CDC[1]

The graph in figure 10 is slightly different from the figure 9. Both of these figures show similar data; however, this figure is slightly blown up so that more details can be seen. In contrast to the figure before this one, you can see how there is a steady increase of cases from 1980 and to around 2000 and then there is a major jump at 2005 and 2010. Just another example of how data presentation can be skewed and misrepresented.

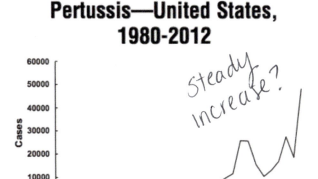

Figure 10. CDC graph showing cases of pertussis in the United States shown from 1980-2012[1]

Varicella = Chix pox

You know what varicella is but by the word "chickenpox". Yes, chickenpox. Yet another sickness people often get when they're children. What's the deal with chickenpox?

This disease is also caused by a virus. It is called the varicella zoster virus and it is a member of the herpesvirus family (yes, herpesvirus). Basically, what that means is that a person can get infected with this virus which is known as the primary infection. After they get better, the virus will live in their body silently until it wants to reap havoc on the body again during a latent infection. The varicella virus can be spread through respiratory transmission or by touching the lesions (the little chickenpox spots). The virus can incubate in the body for 14 to 16 days. For children, the rash appears as the first sign. For adults, there are one to two days of fever and malaise. The body is covered in the rash from the head to the chest and abdomen, to arms, and legs. The rash can also appear in your mucous membranes such as your inner lips or your mouth[1]. It's not a very pleasant experience. The lesions are everywhere and you are very itchy. It can hurt to even try brushing your hair! (Trust me, I know).

The primary infection is known as chickenpox and the reactivation of the latent infection is herpes zoster which is known as shingles[1]. You may have heard of shingles. There are shots advertised for older adults. There's a good reason why. Shingles can be very, very, very painful. Why's that? The varicella zoster virus, after the primary infection, hangs out in sensory nerve ganglia (so in nerve cells). Imagine having an infection in your nerves. Shingles can occur in older adults because of aging, immunosuppression, intrauterine exposure to the virus or having varicella at a young age.

Tetanus

Tetanus is probably one that most people know. In fact, I think most people often associate tetanus with rusty nails. What causes tetanus?

Tetanus is caused by the bacteria *Clostridium tetani*. Interestingly enough, this bacterium can't survive in oxygen so…why exactly are we so concerned about it? The bacteria produce spores, which are kind of like a safe shelter that the bacteria live in until the environment is hospitable enough to live in. The spores are found in soil, the intestines and feces of horses, sheep, cattle, dogs, cats, rats, guinea pigs, and chickens. The spores can also be found on skin and in contaminated heroin[1].

Similar to our lovely bacterial friends that cause diphtheria and pertussis, tetanus is also caused by toxins. This time, there are two toxins that are secreted by the bacteria that we need to worry about. One toxin is called tetanolysin and the other toxin is called tetanospasmin. There isn't exactly a known function for tetanolysin, however, tetanospasmin is a neurotoxin. It's the toxin that causes the known symptoms of the disease[1].

How does the bacteria enter your body? The spores enter through a wound (which is why people associate stepping on a rusty nail with tetanus). The wound obviously does not have to be caused by a rusty nail, it could be anything that allows the spores to enter. Once the spores are inside, the spores will allow the bacteria to grow. These bacteria release the toxins (along with other chemicals). These toxins enter the blood stream and travel to different parts of your central nervous system (which is the brain and spinal cord)[1].

How does this infection progress? It depends on where the person has been infected. The incubation period can be 3 to 21 days. If someone is infected near the central nervous system, there is a shorter incubation time and they are more likely to die. If the infection occurs farther away, there is typically a longer incubation time. In total, there are about three different types of tetanus that can occur. One is known as local tetanus. Another is known as cephalic tetanus and the other one is generalized tetanus. There is also neonatal tetanus that is basically generalized tetanus that occurs in babies that do not have protective passive immunity because the mother was not immune[1].

Local tetanus is uncommon, however, knowing the symptoms and progression can't hurt. When a person experiences local tetanus, there is a persistent contraction of the muscles in the same area where the infection occurred. The contractions may happen for weeks before going away. The infection can also progress to generalized tetanus which is the more common form[1].

In generalized tetanus, there is lockjaw and then neck stiffness. The person has difficulty swallowing and there is abdominal pain. Some other symptoms include an elevated temperature, sweating, elevated blood pressure, and rapid heart rates. There are also spasms. These spasms occur frequently and can last several minutes. The spasms can occur for about three to four weeks and the complete recovery can take months[1].

Cephalic tetanus is very rare. This form has many ear infections. In this form, the bacteria go to the middle ear. The cranial nerves of the face are especially affected in this form.

The complications from tetanus include spasms of the vocal cords, fractures, hypertension, abnormal heart rhythms, nosocomial infections, pulmonary embolisms, aspiration pneumonia, and death[1]. Nosocomial infections are infections that are caused by pathogens in a hospital while pulmonary embolisms are blockages in the arteries to the lungs. An aspiration pneumonia occurs when food, saliva, or stomach acid is inhaled into the lungs.

The treatment for tetanus involved cleaning the wounds and getting rid of any dead tissues. The person may have difficulty breathing so there is a maintenance of the airway. Similar to how the free-floating toxin in diphtheria is removed, the free-floating tetanus toxins are removed through the administration of tetanus immune globulin. After going through all of that, a person still does not have full immunity against tetanus[1].

Tetanus is a disease that is known as very infectious but not contagious. That means that tetanus is essentially a disease that you just need to protect yourself from. There is no chance for you to spread it to another person. Basically, if you get tetanus, you aren't going to hurt anyone else. However, there is a vaccine for it, so why would you want to put yourself at risk for getting tetanus anyway?

The graph from figure 11 shows that cases of tetanus in the United States between 1947 and 2012. The graph shows there was a large decrease in cases around 1970[1]. However, if we zoomed in on this graph, we could probably see a different story. This story could show if there are fluctuations in tetanus cases over the years or if there is just a steady decline.

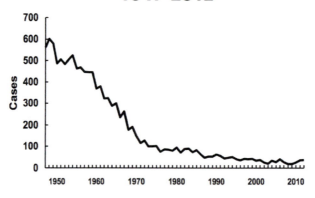

Figure 11. CDC graph depicting the cases of tetanus from 1947 to 2012 [1]

Hepatitis A

Hepatitis A is another disease that you've probably heard of that has a pretty notorious reputation. "Hepatitis" is the inflammation of the liver. The liver is a vital organ in that body. Hepatitis A is caused by a virus. This virus enters the body through a fecal-oral route just like rotavirus and the poliomyelitis virus. Once again, contaminated water, food and poor sanitation are major concerns. Hepatitis A is in the blood and feces for about 10 to 12 days after the infection and can continue to be excreted for up to 3 weeks after the symptoms occur[1].

The symptoms of this disease are fever, malaise, anorexia, nausea, abdominal discomfort, dark urine and jaundice (skin turning yellow). Adults are usually symptomatic whereas children usually do not show any symptoms but are still capable of spreading the disease[1].

For instance, the CDC states that about 70% of the cases that occur in children under the age of 6 are asymptomatic[1]. This statistic means that most young children have the disease and are unknowingly spreading it to the people around them. The virus also stays in the blood after infection which means that it can be spread through transfusions and needles[1].

The complications of this disease involved immunologic, neurologic, hematologic, pancreatic, and renal issues. The main concern of hepatitis A is the development of liver inflammation. There are a few types of liver inflammation such as autoimmune hepatitis, sub-fulminant hepatitis, and fulminant hepatitis[1].

Hepatitis A is still prevalent in Central and South America, Africa, the Middle East, and the Western Pacific. There is no cure or specific treatment for hepatitis A. There are only methods of management. For that reason, vaccinations are the best method of prevention. People traveling to these destinations are given this vaccination. The CDC also recommends all children in the United States should receive this vaccine[1].

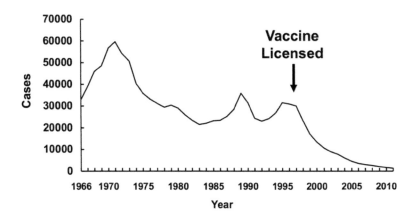

Figure 12. CDC graph depicting the cases of hepatitis A in the United States from 1966 to 2011[1]

The graph in figure 12 show the cases of hepatitis A in 1966 to 2011. The cases of hepatitis were rising and slowly started to decline. The figure indicates that the decline of cases occurred much quicker after the licensure of the vaccine.

These are only some of the infectious diseases that exist in the world. However, all of those diseases have a vaccine that can protect individuals. There are many diseases out in the world that have no vaccine such as Ebola, Zika, HIV, etc. There are also diseases that I didn't mention that have vaccines such as Yellow Fever. Some scientists are working toward making some vaccines toward diseases such as malaria. Other scientists are focused on creating vaccines that prevent and treat cancers.

Luckily, vaccines have been made to prevent a majority of people from contracting these diseases. However, despite how incredibly useful they are, vaccines still have a bad reputation. There are many myths and misinformation that have lead and continue to lead many people astray. For instance, there are people who vehemently believe that vaccines don't work. If they don't work, how have we eradicated smallpox as a disease?

Why are there sudden drops in cases of each disease right after routine vaccination begins? Take a look at figure 2 which shows what happens when people stop vaccinating. The cases of measles were clearly lowered after routine vaccination. When people stopped vaccinating, the cases of measles skyrocketed upward again. Given the evidence, what do you think?

Chapter 3: Do I Have to Get the Flu Shot?

The flu. Everyone hears about the flu. It happens every winter. You see countless signs at pharmacies saying that they have the flu shots. It seems like everyone is saying you should get vaccinated. Why? Isn't it harmless? Why should I get stuck with a needle every year? Do I absolutely have to get this one? What's the deal with the flu?

The flu, or influenza, is caused by a virus. However, there are many types of this virus that exist. There are 4 known types: A, B, C, and D. Types A and B come around and infect people every winter. Type C can infect people and causes respiratory illnesses but does not cause concern for epidemics. The last type, type D, only infects cattle and is not known to infect humans. Another important aspect of these viruses to note is that type A can be found in animals and humans. Whereas types B and C can only be found in humans. Within these four types of virus, there are many more subtypes[1]. For instance, you probably remember when "H1N1" was all over the news in 2009. What does "H1N1" even mean?

The influenza virus has many different forms within the subtypes. The type A has many subtypes that are denoted by the proteins that are present in its shell. The proteins are "hemagglutinin" and "neuraminidase"[2]. Since those are really big words that are also pretty difficult to pronounce, they are just known as "H" and "N" proteins. The number after it describes the different subtype of that protein. For instance, "H1" means that the virus has the hemagglutinin protein of the subtype 1[2]. Below in figure 1, there is a depiction of a generalized influenza virus. There is also a breakdown of how the name of the virus is typically derived.

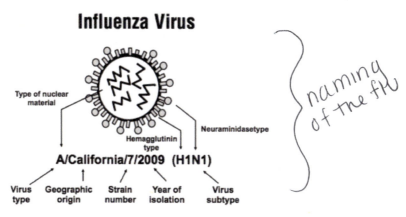

Figure 1. Generalized depiction of influenza virus and naming system from the CDC[2]

Now, let's take a step back. There are four major types of influenza and from those, humans have to be concerned about two of those types. Those two types of virus have two different proteins that each have many different subtypes. There is already a large possibility of combinations that the influenza viruses can be. Then, remember that the type A virus is found in other hosts besides humans. Type A viruses infect other animals such as birds, pigs, and horses. This type is predominantly known to infect waterfowl. Between the many different types of viruses and the different hosts, the influenza virus mutates very often and it is difficult to track.

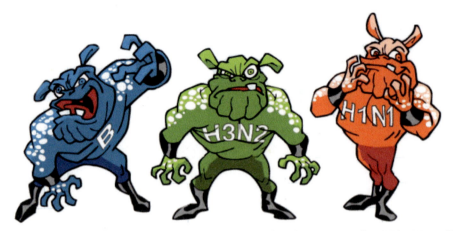

Figure 2. CDC cartoon of the different types of vaccine known as the "Flu Krew"[3]

The flu's symptoms are myalgia (that fancy word for muscle pain!), sore throats, coughing, headaches, and a fever (around 102°-104°)[2]. The flu usually makes people feel so sick that they stay in bed and rest up. A person may also have a runny nose, a burning sensation in their chest and some eye issues (sensitivity to light and eye pain are two examples)[2].

There are also complications associated with the flu just as there are complications with all the other diseases. Some people develop pneumonia after they contract the flu virus. The pneumonia is usually caused by bacteria and is considered a "secondary bacterial pneumonia". The secondary bacterial pneumonia can be caused by bacteria such as *Streptococcus pneumoniae, Haemophilus influenzae,* or *Staphylococcus aureus.* There is also "primary viral pneumonia". This type of pneumonia is very rare and very deadly[2].

Another complication of the flu is Reye syndrome. This syndrome occurs in children who take aspirin when they have been infected with influenza B. The symptoms for Reye syndrome include severe vomiting and confusion. The child is also capable of going into a coma because of brain swelling. For that reason, children and teens are advised not to take aspirin if they are showing flu-like symptoms. Another complication is myocarditis[2].

The other major concern is that the majority of deaths from the flu that occur in the United States are usually with adults over the age of 65 years[2]. That's why there are always signs are pharmacies for people to get the flu. It's really important for people to get protection.

There is a prevalent mindset that the flu isn't very harmful. However, there are always certain populations that are more vulnerable to diseases and the associated complications. As mentioned, older populations are more at risk. Younger children are also at risk for dangerous complications. It's really not "just the flu".

>*higher risk populations*

Historically speaking, the flu has had very scary moments. One of the deadliest pandemics occurred in 1918[4]. Side note, the word "pandemic" refers to an outbreak of a disease that occurs around world while the word "epidemic" refers to an outbreak that can occurs on a smaller scale.

In 1918, the Spanish Influenza pandemic took the lives of around 50 million people[4]. Meanwhile, it was estimated that about 50% of the world was infected with this disease[5]. This pandemic was caused by a strain of the H5N1[4]. It was so serious that scientists and researchers are still trying to figure out how it spread so quickly. In fact, the CDC, the U.S. Department of Agriculture, National Institutes of Health, and Armed Forces Institutes of Pathology all worked together to try to reconstruct and figure out what exactly happened in that flu pandemic[6].

Fast-forward, you may remember this, in 2009, the world saw the H1N1 flu pandemic. Personally, I remember many people were very concerned during this time period. For instance, the WHO declared the H1N1 epidemic as a pandemic on June 11, 2009. A few months later, sometime around December 5, 2009, 208 countries around the world reported over 10,000 deaths combined[7]. After the pandemic, there were 18,500 laboratory-confirmed deaths[8]. This number may not even be representative of the actual pandemic as there may not have been autopsies that detected the flu virus in some bodies. Definitely not as large as the 50 million deaths of 1918 but that is still an insane number of deaths. Since this was one of the more recent pandemics, there is still ongoing research regarding this pandemic.

But that was in 2009, there had to have been more medical advances since then, right? Let' think about the more recent outbreaks. The flu season beginning in October of 2017 and moving into 2018 was pretty brutal. During this time, the flu shot is always widely advertised. However, the shot didn't account for all the strains that were occurring that season. No one should really be to blame. Scientists can have misjudgments too, after all, everyone is human. Don't believe me? The figures below show the different types of influenza that were prevalent throughout 2017 and 2018. The graph in figure 3 shows the different strains that were common in North America. There were mostly influenza types A that were not subtyped as the dark blue indicates.

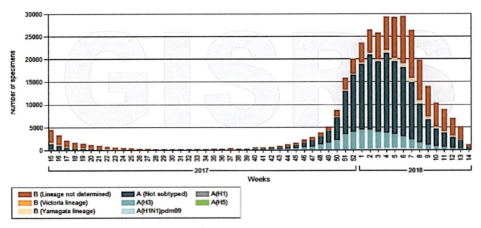

Figure 3. Influenza specimens by subtype in North America from WHO Update in April 2018 [2]

In the following graph in figure 4, eastern Asia shows different types were popular throughout the year. For this region of the world, there seemed to be more of the type A(H3) for most of 2017. In the following months, type B of the Yamagata lineage was more popular along with type A (H1N1). Compared to North America, there were certainly different strains that were more prevalent but between the two there were also type B of unknown lineages that were prevalent.

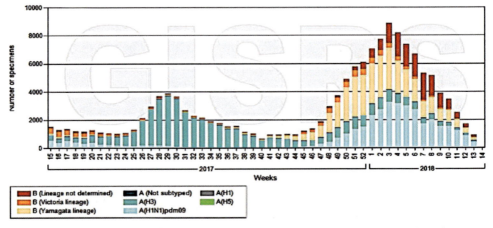

Figure 4. Influenza specimens by subtype in Eastern Asia from WHO Update in April 2018 [2]

The following graph, figure 5, shows the different subtypes of the southern hemisphere. Notice how these countries experienced the flu season earlier in 2017. Remember, the winter in the southern hemisphere happens during the summer of the northern hemisphere. This graph shows similar strains as figure 4 with the subtypes found in North America. However, there were more cases of the A (H3) than the unknown type B in this region of the world.

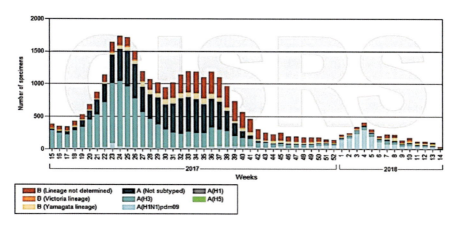

Figure 5. Influenza specimens by subtype in the Southern Hemisphere from WHO Update in April 2018 [2]

As those graphs can show, there were many types of influenza that were infecting people all around the world. No one wonder the season lasted for so long. Also, the graphs show how difficult it could be for scientists to create a vaccine that could protect against all the types that may potentially be prevalent. In terms of the big picture, would you rather get a vaccine with say 40% protection or have 0% protection?

Now, I want to shift gears just a little bit. Sure enough, the flu is terrible and the vaccine is available. The question is, what do people think of it? There is one super prominent myth out there. The myth is the following: The flu vaccine gave me the flu. *myth* Let's go over that a little bit. As mentioned an earlier chapter, the routine influenza vaccine contains a killed virus. The nasal spray has the live attenuated virus which is very different from the injection. The killed virus vaccine is what is injected through an intramuscular route (so into your muscle). The antigen is killed. It cannot replicate. It cannot mutate. It cannot give someone the flu. *IM injection*

Why does it hurt to get the shot? Why do some people claim they got the flu? For the first question, the needle is going into the arm muscles which can lead to soreness. Sometimes, the administrator may go too deep into the muscle or just do it wrong. Sometimes, the soreness is a result from the antigen acting with the immune system.

For the second question, some people do feel a little sick after the vaccine. This reaction is normal. The vaccine is injected which means the antigen has been put into the body. This antigen has to work with your immune system to create the antibody response. If you feel a little sick afterwards, that may just be your body reacting to the antigen and creating an immune response to protect you. If you are still convinced you have the flu, think about your symptoms. Are you so sick that you are experiencing myalgia? Do you have a fever? What about a sore throat? Are you coughing? Do you have light sensitivity? Oh, and this is the most important question: Did you see a doctor? Or are you just self-diagnosing (Don't feel bad, yours truly also self-diagnoses like a fool but ends up with the doctor for a professional opinion).

Overall, the influenza vaccine needs to be given every year. The reason for this is because there are different flu strains that are popular every year. As a result, scientists try to study and figure out which strains they think will probably be the most prevalent in the upcoming season. Ultimately, the flu vaccine is a concoction of educated guesses. It may not be perfect but some protection is certainly better than zero protection.

For that reason, the vaccine may not be able to protect people against every strain that occurs. There may be a season, such as recently, where there is a strain that occurs that was not in the flu vaccine. That's why every year, health care professionals recommend getting the flu vaccine. It's sort of like getting an update with your phone. The new one comes out and you download it (some people may delay it, but you know you shouldn't). The same goes for the flu vaccine. Every season, a new vaccine comes out and you should go get the new one.

As mentioned, this vaccine since it isn't exactly required in most places and you are actively asking someone to stick a needle in your body. For that reason, there are many people who avoid getting the shot. They are just afraid of needles. There is nothing wrong with that. However, the bottom line is that the vaccine is important and it protects you and the people around you. After all, it's not just the flu.

Chapter 4: Meningitis

You wake up one Monday morning. It's 9am. You went out all weekend with your friends so you just spent your entire Sunday night working on that English paper. You know, that same paper you were assigned the first week of classes but you decided to procrastinate. You managed to get to bed at 5am and all you want to do is sleep but your first class is at 10am. You roll yourself out of bed. You feel sick and tired. It's probably just because you were up late last night. You get yourself to class and you start feeling more lethargic. Your body is beginning to ache so you decide you'll go to the health center when your class is over. However, you're sitting in class and you find it difficult to listen to your professor talk because you're just so exhausted. Class is finally over and you walk over to the health center. You don't even know how you made that trek because your back hurts. The nurses there check you out and assure you that you only have the flu so they send you back to your dorm and tell you to sleep it off. You decide to miss the rest of your classes so you can take your recovery nap. Not even half an hour into your nap, your roommate comes and wakes you up.

Normally, this wouldn't bother you but as you get up, you realize your ankles feel like they're bleeding. You check under the blankets and there's a rash forming. It looks strangely purple and you don't know what's wrong. You still feel like you got hit by a bus and you tell your roommate. Your roommate calls the RA over and the next thing you know is that you're in a hospital bed. What happened? You look around. Your parents are next to you. You hear someone crying. You have no idea why you were there. It was only the flu…or was it? It turns out you were in a medically induced coma for at least a week while the doctors were frantically trying to keep you alive. What happened?

In this scenario, you had contracted bacterial meningitis during your wild weekend. Meningitis is an inflammation of the meninges which are a tissue that protect your brain and your spinal cord. As you can imagine, the meninges are incredibly important in keeping your body protected. There are many different causes of meningitis. Typically, bacteria and viruses cause meningitis infections. There are other causes, however, in regards to the purpose of this book, one specific bacterial meningitis is the focus.

The bacterial meningitis that you experienced in the hypothetical situation is known as meningococcal meningitis. This type of meningitis is caused by the bacteria known as *Nesseria meningitidis.* There are twelve known serotypes of this bacteria. Of those twelve types, there are six that have been known to cause epidemics and they are the following: A, B, C, W, X and Y[1]. In the United States, the CDC recommends that everyone gets the meningococcal vaccine. The CDC has recommended children receive this vaccine at the ages of 11 and 12. However, if they receive this vaccination at this age, they may need a booster at 16. For people who receive the vaccine at 16, there is no need to get a booster for the MenACWY vaccine[7]. The vaccine that is given typically contains four of the six strains that cause meningococcal meningitis. The strains that are covered

[Margin note: vaccine for Strain B released later]

in this vaccine are: A, C, W and Y. According to the CDC, the most recent outbreaks, as of 2015, are caused by the B, C, and Y strains. However, notice how the vaccine that is recommended only provides protection against strains A, C, W, and Y. If strain B has been a cause of recent outbreaks, why aren't people getting vaccinated for it? The vaccine was not available as it was not released until sometime in late 2014[1]. This vaccine was difficult to produce because the serogroup B has two more subtypes beyond that. For that reason, many people are not vaccinated against this disease and the CDC only began recommending it in 2015.

What exactly happens when someone is infected with *N. meningitidis*? Let's begin when a person gets infected. The bacteria incubate in the body for about three to four days[1]. This disease is interesting because health care professionals can categorize the symptoms into two subcategories.

As mentioned, the bacteria can infect meninges and cause meningitis. If the bacteria enter the bloodstream, it is called meningococcemia. The symptoms of meningitis include neck stiffness, sensitivity to bright light, seizures, and severe headaches. The symptoms of just meningococcemia are the purplish rash, unusually cold hands and feet, fast breathing and breathlessness and limb, joint and muscle pain[5]. For both of these progressions, the person can feel very sleepy, have a high fever, experience vomiting, and be confused/delirious. In most cases, the person will have both meningitis and meningococcemia so there is a combination of those symptoms[5]. The speed at which these symptoms greatly vary between people. This infection also spreads very, very quickly. The figure below is from the NMA and is a very simple and clear depiction of the symptoms[5].

[Margin note: most people have both]

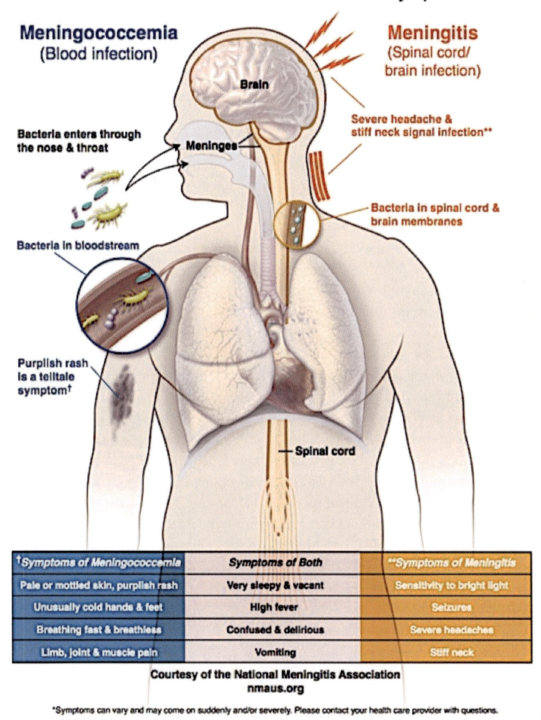

Figure 1. Diagram from NMA showing simplified symptoms of meningitis[5]

So, how exactly does this disease even infect someone in the first place? Humans are the only known carriers so your furry friends are not likely to give you meningococcal meningitis. In the human population, according to the NMA, about one in ten people carry the meningococcal bacteria in their noses or throats without showing any symptoms or signs[3]. These people are capable of spreading the disease and not even know it. The bacteria spreads through respiratory secretions and close contact such as kissing[6]. However, it can also spread through sneezing and coughing[6].

Why should college students care about meningococcal meningitis? The answer is pretty simple. College students are at a high risk for contracting the bacteria and spreading it to each other[4]. In the United States, there are 600 to 1000 cases of meningococcal meningitis each year[3]. Of those cases, 10 to 15% of those people die because of the disease[3]. Another important point to note is that in the United States, 21% of the cases involve people between the ages of 11 and 24[3]. Yes, that's right, preteens, teens, and young adults are all at very high risk. As mentioned, college students are particularly at a high risk. Why's that?

Remember, college dorm buildings house many students. For the most part, there are common bathrooms and shared dorm rooms. For instance, my freshman year, I lived in a normal sized dorm room with three other girls. We shared a common bathroom with half the floor. If any of the girls on the floor contracted meningitis, it would be a great environment for the disease to spread. College students are put in an ideal environment for different diseases to spread. For that reason, I would suggest bringing some fever and cough medications. There is a pretty good chance that you are going to get sick a few times during your first year at school (even if you are commuting).

The map below shows the number of meningococcal cases on college campuses in the United States between 2013 and 2017[8]. Some of these students were able to survive, for instance, looking at the orange box below "2013-2017", one can see that Penn State University had two cases that survived[8]. Right next to it, UMASS Amherst had two cases that survived but these survivals were during an outbreak. Just below that though, you can see there was one death at Northeastern University. The cases at Penn State and Northeastern were non-serogroup B whereas the cases at UMASS Amherst were confirmed as serogroup B[8]. Looking at other colleges, there was a student who died at Dakota-Wesleyan University of non-serogroup B type[8]. This infection is very real. It's not some made up story. There are outbreaks that occur sporadically. This map shows real college students who became the statistics that were mentioned earlier.

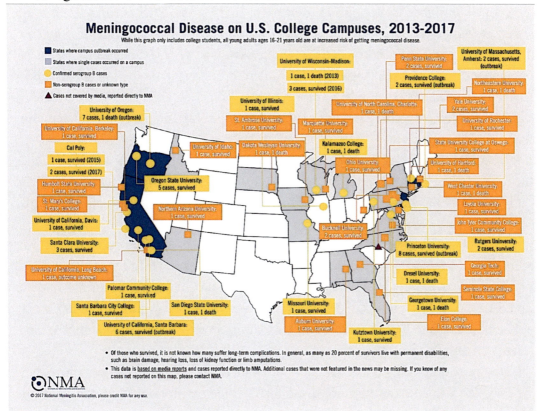

Figure 2. Map of meningococcal disease on U.S. college campuses from NMA[8]

Now in the hypothetical situation, the doctors put you into a coma for a week. During that time period, you were at risk for losing parts of your body. The infection had spread so quickly that the doctors had to amputate your right arm. Don't believe me?

According to Ireland's Health Service Executive, some complications from meningococcal meningitis include: hearing loss (either partial or total), issues with memory and concentration, issues with balance and coordination, speech problems, and vision loss (partial or total). A major complication for some patients is caused by gangrene. During the meningococcal infection that travels through the blood, the bacteria can kill body tissues[8]. As a result, physicians perform amputations of any body parts such as fingers and limbs that have been infected[8]. For that reason, your arm was amputated in the hypothetical scenario.

In order for someone to get the meningococcal meningitis diagnosis, they need to undergo a series of tests. These tests involve obtaining a culture from the patient before antibiotics are administered[1]. If antibiotics are administered, a blood sample, cerebrospinal fluid/CSF (a liquid that protects your spine and brain), or other specimens can be tested using PCR[1]. PCR stands for polymerase chain reaction. PCR is a method that takes a small amount of nucleic acids such as DNA or RNA and amplifies it (makes multiple copies) until there is enough for detection. In this case, PCR is run to determine if there is *N. meningitidis*. There are also kits that facilitate a rapid and specific way of detecting the bacteria[1]. These kits test the CSF for antigens. This test is specifically used for meningococcal serotype B. The CSF is obtained through spinal taps[1]. A spinal tap is basically when a needle is stuck into a spine and the fluid is obtained. As you can see, getting the vaccine and avoiding meningococcal meningitis is much easier than actually contracting the disease.

If you think I'm making all of this up to scare you, I suggest you watch this video from the NMA linked right here: https://youtu.be/jjIY0XTzsn0[12]. If you didn't watch the video, it is basically the story of a girl who was about to go to college and did not get the vaccine.

She is living evidence that anyone can contract a disease. Race, gender, socioeconomic status, sexuality, none of that matters. A disease will infect anyone. There are no boundaries. Kaitlyn got sick. The scary part, she was just another normal student going to college. She made the decision not to get vaccinated. She probably didn't want another needle stuck into her arm and felt it was unimportant. However, she almost died from learning that was a mistake.

If you're still thinking about taking your chances and skipping out on this vaccination when you get your immunization forms filled out, I would suggest you watch this video from the NMA next: https://youtu.be/ASg5Pef4WuM[13].

Now, if you didn't watch this video, it's the story of a girl whose mom buried her in her prom dress. This girl was a senior in high school. She also got infected and got very ill. In her case, she didn't survive. Her family had to make a tough decision. They had to bury her. She never got to finish high school. She never got to go to college. She was robbed of so many opportunities all because of tiny bacteria. Don't end up like her. You have all the opportunities that she couldn't have. You should consider yourself incredibly lucky.

The bottom line is that this vaccine is important and can protect you. There may be students at your university who decided not to get vaccinated. For all you know, someone may be carrying that bacteria in their nose and sneeze on you. Or maybe you go out to a club and someone nearby is coughing. Or you aren't the partying type, but you live in a cramped residence hall. The question is simple: would you rather have a needle poked into your arm or have your arm amputated?

Chapter 5: Let's Talk Sex.

Yep, I said it. Sex. Now, I'm not here to tell you whether you should be having sex, or who to have sex with or how to have sex. All of those details are up to you. You can very well decide you don't want to be sexually active when you first begin college. You may very well decide that you want to be very sexually active. You may decide that you want to be in a committed monogamous relationship. You may decide you want to stay single and avoid all sexual activity. Or, you may decide you want to be in fluid and polygamous relationships. Those are your details to worry about and not the focus of this chapter.

Regardless of whether you are partaking or what you believe, sex is a major component of life, especially college life. For instance, there may be one Friday night while you're innocently watching Netflix and eating ice cream in bed. And then, suddenly, you hear thumping and moans upstairs and you realize, yep, the girl upstairs is having sex. (My advice for this situation: TURN THAT NETFLIX UP. This advice works if you are the girl having sex or if you are me in this situation ;)).

Or, you may be getting ready for a night out. While you're checking yourself out in the mirror, you get a text from that cutie in your English class. All you can think about is how you can't wait to go home with them tonight. (I also hope you remember the condoms, those are very important). Maybe you're sitting in class and your professor starts a discussion on human sexuality begins. Or you're walking around campus and you see a flyer for a Sex Ed event hosted by your one of your school's many organizations. You may even simply be having a conversation about sex with your roommates. No matter what, the topic of sex will come up. So why am I making this a big deal?

Sex is fun. However, along with that fun, there are some serious consequences that can arise from being irresponsible. I'm not just talking about getting pregnant. (But yes, pregnancy is still something to worry about if you're sexually active). When people engage in sex, there are many bodily fluids that come in contact. Naturally, human bodies have lots of microorganisms. Many of those are not harmful. However, there are many out there that can do more harm than you realize.

At this point in your life, if you've had the uncomfortable "Sex Ed" class in your high school health class or a serious discussion with your parents, you probably know what I'm about to say.

STDS. Yes. Sexually Transmitted Diseases. Many of which you may have heard of such as gonorrhea, chlamydia, HIV/AIDS, HPV, and hepatitis. Many of these diseases sound super scary. They're undesirable. No college student wants to get those. Actually, it doesn't matter if you're in college or not. No one wants a sexually transmitted disease. The reality is that some of your peers may be carrying these diseases. They may be aware. They may not be aware. If you are sexually active or you want to become sexually active, you may want to take the time to educate yourself a little further and take some precautions.

Let's begin by discussing the term "sexual activity." The term isn't very clear. "Sexual activity" encompasses all behaviors that are considered sexual. I mean it, ALL behaviors. These behaviors could be kissing, oral sex, anal sex, vaginal sex and everything in between. Most of the time, when people refer to sexual activity, they are only thinking about sexual intercourse. ==Viruses and bacteria spread through any type of sexual activity that involves physical contact==. It doesn't matter if you only engage in oral sex or strictly vaginal sex. The pathogens can spread through any way. Since most people only refer to "sex" as "vaginal sex," they think that oral sex or anal sex can be safer. Don't be fooled by that misconception. At any point, when one body part is in contact with another without any physical barrier, pathogens can spread from one person to another.

For that reason, protection is very important. In the moment you might think, one risky night can't be that bad. However, in that one instance, you could contract a disease that you could have for the rest of your life. Why not just be safe from the beginning and avoid contracting, say, gonorrhea or chlamydia?

In terms of protection, there are a variety of ways to prevent pregnancy, that will not protect against STDs. There are also methods that people use to prevent pregnancy that are very risky and not fully effective. Let's address those, shall we?

Withdrawal. (A.K.A. The Pull-Out Method). Yes, there are many people in the world who use the pull-out method to avoid pregnancy. However, what happens someone doesn't pull out in time? It's not a reliable method of preventing pregnancy. It is also does not protect from any STDs because there is skin-to-skin contact. In this scenario, fluids are still interacting with different body parts and the diseases have easy access[4].

Birth control implant. The birth control implant is for females. It is a little rod that is placed in the body and releases hormones that prevent pregnancy. This method is 99% effective in preventing pregnancies. However, this method alone provides 0% protection against STDs[4].

Birth control pill. The pills are only going to protect women from pregnancy. The pill also has to be taken at the same time every day to be protective. This method is only 91% protective. They will not protect against STDs since there is no physical barrier between secretions and body parts[4].

Birth control patch. This is a little patch that is placed on any part of your body. It releases hormones that are absorbed by the skin. The patch is also like the pill and is 91% effective in protecting against pregnancy. This method also provides no protection against STDs[4].

Birth control shots. This form of birth control is a hormonal shot given every 3 months by a health care professional. It is 94% effective at preventing pregnancies. However, this method also has zero protection against STDs[4].

Birth control sponge. The birth control sponge is a piece of soft and squishy plastic. It is placed deep inside the vagina. It also has a spermicide. The sponge can also be placed inside the vagina 24 hours before sex and there is a little loop that can be pulled on to remove it. This form of birth control is 76 to 88% effective. It does not protect against STDs. In fact, one disadvantage is that is can actually promote the growth of STDs[4].

Birth control vaginal ring. This ring uses hormones just like the birth control pill to stop eggs from being released. The ring is worn inside the vagina so the lining absorbs the hormones. The ring can be placed in the vagina for the month. It is 91% effective and does not protect against STDs[4].

Cervical cap. This is a little piece of silicone that is placed deep inside the vagina. It looks like a sailor's cap and covers the cervix so that way sperm doesn't get to the egg. However, this form of birth control is only 86% for women who haven't given birth and 71% effective for women who have given birth. The cap has to be used correctly and must stay there for at least 6 hours after sex. Adding spermicide makes it more effective at protecting against pregnancy. The cervical cap does not protect against STDs either[4].

Diaphragm. The diaphragm is similar to the cervical cap. The shape is different because instead of looking like a sailor's cap, it looks like a little saucer. It's basically a very shallow cup made of silicon that needs to be bent in half and then placed in the vagina to cover the cervix. They are 94% effective if used perfectly every time. More realistically, it is 88% effective. Diaphragms also work more effectively if a spermicide is used along with it. Just like the other forms of birth control, diaphragms do not work to protect against STDs[4].

Spermicide. This method of birth control works by two methods. It can block the cervix so sperm doesn't get in. It can also stop the sperm form moving. Spermicide can be a foam, a gel, a film, a cream or a soft insert that melts into a cream in the vagina. Spermicide can be 71% effective. This form of birth control also does not protect against STDs. In fact, it can increase the risk of getting a STD. How? Spermicides have a chemical that can cause the vagina to get irritated and makes it easier for pathogens to enter the body[4].

IUDs. These are also only going to protect women from pregnancy. What's an IUD? The abbreviation sort of makes it sound like an STD, right? IUD stands for intrauterine device. This method of birth control is when a tiny T-shaped piece of plastic or metal is placed in the cervix. There are two types of IUDs. There are hormonal IUDs that release hormones in the body. There are also copper IUDs. These work by killing off sperm because copper is a spermicide. IUDs are 99% protective when it comes to pregnancies. Copper IUDs can also be placed inside the cervix after unsafe sex if someone is worried about pregnancy. When the IUD is placed after unsafe sex, it is 99% effective at preventing the pregnancy. However, in terms of STDs, they also do not provide a physical barrier between fluids and body parts[4].

I hope by now you're sensing a pattern. All of the above are methods that females can use to prevent pregnancy. If you're a male, you should probably also keep the various types in mind. The information isn't going to hurt you and you could give someone helpful advice. All of these methods are pretty effective at preventing pregnancy. However, STDs are capable of spreading no matter which form you use. There is one recommendation that is suggested to be used along with any of the above birth control methods. You can probably guess it considering it's very well-known.

Condoms. That's right. Condoms are the only method that can help protect against STDs. Most people know about male condoms. There are also female condoms. Male condoms and female condoms, when used correctly, can protect against pregnancy and STDs[4]. Male condoms are the more commonly used. However, they have to be used correctly. There can't be any holes. They can't be reused. (I'm just putting that out there in case anyone thought otherwise…). Also, make sure that it's put on correctly. Remember the banana demonstrations?

In an ideal world, all methods of protection, whether it be helmets, vaccines, or condoms, would be 100% protective. However, the world isn't ideal. Things are imperfect. There is always a chance that something could go wrong. So even if you used a condom, there is still a chance it could break. Or maybe it had a hole before you even opened it (I remember watching some people do the Condom Challenge and it turned out the condom they were using had a hole in it. Yikes!)

In terms of all the birth control methods that have been mentioned, condoms are the only method that protect against STDs. It is the only method that provides a physical barrier between skin and fluids. However, they're only 85% effective. The other issue is that condoms do not cover all the areas that could transmit a STD to a person. For instance, herpes can be spread through skin to skin contact. If someone touches a part where the condom isn't covering, there's a very high chance that a STD can spread.

In terms of oral sex, mouth to genital contact will spread many different germs just like vaginal sex or anal sex. In fact, chlamydia, gonorrhea, and herpes can all spread through oral sex. It can be spread whether you are receiving and giving. The good news is that there is treatment for chlamydia and gonorrhea. If chlamydia and gonorrhea go untreated, it can cause infertility issues for women[6].

Now let's talk some specific diseases. There aren't many vaccines when it comes to sexually transmitted diseases. Even if there are some vaccines, they're considered highly controversial. At this moment let's talk about some very specific and well-known STDs.

Chlamydia infects both males and females. It can be spread through oral, vaginal, and anal sex. An exchange of fluids does not have to occur for the disease to spread between two people. If someone were to get chlamydia and receive treatment, they are still at risk for getting it again. As mentioned, chlamydia is serious when it is left untreated. It can damage the female reproductive system and make it difficult to get pregnant later in life. It can also cause ectopic pregnancies which is a pregnancy that occurs outside of the womb[1].

As mentioned there is treatment for chlamydia. The treatment has to be completed and it cannot be shared. The treatment is typically a series of antibiotics for seven days[7]. A person is also advised not to have sex while taking the treatment to avoid spreading the disease to other people[7]. What are the symptoms? For women, there is a burning sensation when urinating and an abnormal vaginal discharge. For men, there is a penile discharge, also a burning sensation when urinating, and pain and swelling in the testicles. There is also the possibility of rectal pain, discharge and bleeding if anal sex was involved[1]. The infections may not be noticeable but those are the possible symptoms. Just as a side note, a pregnant woman can also give her baby chlamydia. That baby could experience an eye infection and develop pneumonia[1].

Gonorrhea infects both men and women as well[8]. In the United States, there is an estimated 820,000 new cases of N. gonorrhoeae infections each year[10]. According to the CDC, there are an estimated 2.86 million cases of gonorrhea that occurs annually[8]. It spreads through anal, oral, and vaginal sex[8].

There is treatment for gonorrhea, however, it is getting more difficult to treat. The recommended treatment for gonorrhea is a dual therapy[9]. This therapy requires a dose of intramuscular ceftriaxone and one dose of oral azithromycin. That is one shot and one pill (which doesn't just happen once)[9]. There are also causes of antimicrobial drug resistant gonorrhea[9]. What that means is that the disease can't be treated as the microorganism isn't killed by the medicines. These resistant microorganisms begin to exist as more people use antimicrobials and antibiotics more often. Just as the treatment for chlamydia shouldn't be shared, the treatment for gonorrhea shouldn't be shared either.

Most men or women do not show the symptoms of gonorrhea. However, the symptoms of gonorrhea for men are the following: burning sensation while urinating, a white/yellow/green penile discharge, and painful or swollen testicles[8]. For women, the symptoms are the following: painful/burning sensation while urinating, increased vaginal discharge, and vaginal bleeding in between periods[8]. Similar to chlamydia, rectal infections can also occur but are not likely. The following are symptoms of a rectal infection: discharge, anal itching, soreness, bleeding, and painful bowel movements[8]. Just as chlamydia can be given to a baby, gonorrhea can also be given to a baby at birth.

Hepatitis A was already discussed in the VPDs chapter so I will also talk about hepatitis C along with it. Hepatitis A can be spread sexually. It is not limited to just the oral-fecal route. According to the CDC, condoms are not very effective at protecting against hepatitis A. The best way to protect oneself from the disease is literally just from being vaccinated. Onto hepatitis C! Hepatitis C is pretty scary because there is no vaccine for it. It typically is not spread through sexual activity. However, it is still very possible to get hepatitis C. This disease is blood-borne so needle-sticks are typically the major concern. Hepatitis C can cause fatal liver damage. A person can develop chronic hepatitis after infection and of those people 70% will develop active liver disease. From there around 10 to 20% develop liver cirrhosis and then 1 to 5% develop liver cancer[17].

Herpes is a little more complicated than the other diseases that have been covered thus far. A person can get genital herpes or oral herpes. The viruses are called the herpes simplex viruses and there are two types of this virus. They are abbreviated as HSV-1 and HSV-2[11]. Oral herpes is only caused by HSV-1[11]. It causes cold sores or fever blisters around or on the mouth. Most people do not have the symptoms. They typically contract this virus through non-sexual activity when they are young children. It happens because of contact with saliva[11].

The HSV-1, the one that causes oral herpes, can spread to the genitals through oral sex which is where the STD portion comes in. In terms of prevalence, the CDC states that "more than one out of every six people aged 14 to 49 have genital herpes". To me, that's a pretty large number of people. How does it spread? As like the other STDS, it can spread through oral, anal and vaginal sex. A herpes sore is typically what will spread the disease to another person. Saliva and genital secretions will also spread the disease. The disease will spread with skin contact to either oral or genital infections[11].

If a person gets infected, they typically do not realize that they have genital herpes. The first time a person has an "outbreak" can be confusing as they may have flu-like symptoms and the skin lesions may look like another condition. Going to a doctor will help as they can diagnose you. If they perform a blood test, they won't be able to tell who infected you or how long you've had it though. Now, the sad part, there is no cure for herpes. There are medications to prevent outbreaks from happening or shorten them. This treatment includes anti-herpes medication that can be taken daily which makes it less likely it will spread to a partner. If a person doesn't get treated, the genital herpes will probably hurt. If you touch the sores and fluids, it can spread to other parts of the body. As I've given information about pregnancy about the other diseases, there is also information about herpes and pregnancy. A pregnancy woman can give her child herpes during birth and it cause a deadly disease labeled as "neonatal herpes". These women have to work very closely with their doctors to determine the best course of action for their babies[11].

Moving onto another very well-known STD. Human Immunodeficiency Virus which is also known as HIV. HIV has a pretty horrifying and sad history in terms of public health in the United States. However, this book is only going to cover the symptoms, treatment, and transmission of HIV. By now, you know the drill. It can be spread through oral, anal, and vaginal sex. It spreads through bodily fluids which include blood semen, vaginal fluids, rectal fluids, and breast milk[4]. So, a person can also get it from non-sexual activities such as intravenous drug use (otherwise known as injecting drugs)[18]. Basically, if it's a fluid coming out of the body (of an infected person), it contains HIV. There are no reliable symptoms that a person can use to figure out if they have HIV. They need to get tested[13].

What does HIV do? The virus destroys specific cells in the human system which is why it is so dangerous. There is no cure for HIV. Once a person has it, they have to take a treatment for it every single day. These drugs are known as ART or antiretroviral therapy[12]. The drugs have to be taken every single day. Compliance (keeping up with the medicines) may difficult as it has to be taken every day. The drug basically keeps the viral load (the amount of virus in the blood) at lower levels. There are more treatments options that are being highly researched but ARTs are the best treatment as of now. If you are someone who knows you will be encountering HIV, then you can also take a precautionary step and take PrEP. PrEP stands for "pre-exposure prophylaxis"[14]. This treatment is basically a combination of two medicines that can lower the chance of a person getting HIV[14]. This drug also has to be taken consistently in order to work.

If there is also a chance that someone thinks that they have been exposed to HIV, they can take PEP which stands for "post-exposure prophylaxis"[15]. It has to be taken within three days and is taken daily for four weeks in order to prevent an HIV infection[15]. In terms of people who are infected, the disease can progress to more serious conditions if they do not comply to their medications. They can progress through the three stages of the disease. The first stage is known as the acute HIV infection[12]. The second stage is known as clinical latency. The final stage is AIDS which stands for "acquired immunodeficiency syndrome"[12].

Another important point to note is that there are different types of HIV viruses that exist. Some people can get infected with multiple types and they are known to have a "superinfection"[12]. Before the medications, HIV and AIDS were deadly. If a person found out they had contracted HIV, it was a death sentence. Luckily, there is more research now and there are options available today.

Syphilis can also be spread by the ways that we have already mentioned. It can cause some serious health complications. Syphilis is a little different from the other diseases as there can be four stages to this disease. The disease can be the following: primary, secondary, latent, and tertiary. The primary stage has sores that occur where the infection first entered the body. The sores are painless and last from 3 to 6 weeks regardless of treatment. The secondary stage is when skin rashes or mucous membrane lesions or both show. These skin rashes and lesions aren't going to be painful either. They will be brown-ish or red. They can also show up as the primary stage fades away. Other symptoms of this stage include fever, swollen lymph glands, sore throat, patchy hair loss, headaches, weight loss, muscles aches and fatigue. The latent stage is when a person has no symptoms but they still carry the disease and can spread it to other people[16].

The final stage only occurs when people do not get treatment. When this stage occurs, the disease starts infecting other organ systems. It can infect the heart, blood vessels, and nervous system. This stage occurs 10 to 30 years after the initial syphilis infection. The damage to the organs can cause death. For each of these stages, there is treatment and treatment can stop the disease from progressing. The treatment is through the antibiotics that are specifically prescribed for the disease. The treatment cannot undo any damage that has already been done to the body (similar to gonorrhea). For pregnant women, syphilis can infect an unborn baby. The baby is likely to have a low-birth weight. There is also a strong possibility of a premature delivery or stillborn[16].

Among these STDs, there are a few that can be prevented through vaccination. Hepatitis B and the Human Papillomavirus (HPV) are both preventable diseases! These are both commonly known diseases. How about we take a look into these diseases?

Hep B

Let's start with hepatitis B because this vaccine is given to children in the United States almost immediately after they are born. As mentioned earlier, hepatitis is the inflammation of the liver and there are multiple ways for this to occur in humans. Hepatitis B is a disease caused by a hepadnaviridae virus[1]. Hepatitis B, like the other hepatitis diseases, cause inflammation of the liver. This specific disease is of major importance because of prevalence. It is also very easy to transmit through sexual behavior which is different from the other two hepatitis viruses[17]. Hepatitis B can also be passed through injected drug use. The disease also passes through to babies at birth[1].

Most people who have hepatitis B do not realize they have the disease because symptoms typically do not show. However, if symptoms do show they are usually fever, fatigue, loss of appetite, nausea, vomiting, dark urine, grey stool, joint paint, and jaundice (yellowing skin and eyes). In terms of the infection, there can be an acute hepatitis B infection or a chronic hepatitis B infection. The acute infection occurs in the first 6 months after the initial infection. There is usually no illness or a mild form of the illness. A person can get the infection and clear it and be immune to the hepatitis B virus. In terms of the chronic hepatitis B infection, a person gets the disease and has it for the rest of their life. This type of infection typically happens with babies. They develop the chronic infection which over time can cause the fatal liver damage, cirrhosis, liver cancer and eventually death[1]. For that reason, babies are typically given the vaccine right at birth so they are capable of being protected immediately.

HPV

HPV stands for human papillomavirus. Many young females may have heard of this STD when their pediatricians offered the Gardasil vaccination. What exactly is HPV? HPV is a virus that can cause genital warts, cancers and other health issues. There are over 100 types of HPV in existence[21]. Some of these types cause cancers. Others are not as harmful and often can cause genital warts. These warts can be small or large, raise or flat and sometimes look like cauliflower. The HPV that causes warts do not cause cancer [19]. A medical professional can certainly look at the warts and let you know if you are ever in the position to figure it out. In terms of prevalence, according to the CDC, there are an estimated 79 million people who are infected in the United States. It is also estimated that there are 14 million new cases of HPV infections that occur every year and about half of those people are between the ages of 15 and 24[1].

When the vaccine for HPV was created, it was marketed as a way to prevent cervical cancer. Since only females have cervixes, the vaccine was offered only to females. However, males are fully capable of being infected. The odd part is that males were not recommended to receive this vaccine. However, if an infected woman were to have sex with a man. That man is going to be infected and he may decide to have sex with another woman who was not initially infected. Why did they decide that only women needed protection and men didn't? All of those sexual relationships are also only accounting for heterosexual relationships. What happens in more fluid relationships?

Don't be fooled by people who say "most infections go away on their own, you don't need the vaccine." They are not wrong. Many infections that are caused by HPV can go away on their own. However, as mentioned earlier, there are many types of HPV. Some types are not that harmful and the symptoms can go away. However, you are still going to be carrying this virus and you can spread it to other people. The other issue is that the vaccine protects against the more dangerous types of HPV. The first vaccine that was made was marketed as "Cervarix" because it prevented cervical cancer. This vaccine only had protection against two types of HPV, 16 and 18[1]. This vaccine was also marketed only for females. Why? Here was the logic. It protects against cervical cancer and males don't have cervixes. If they don't have cervixes, they can't get that cancer. (MASSIVE FACEPALM.)

Remember, microorganisms don't care who you are. You are a warm, human body. You have lots of nutrients and you provide the ideal environment for them to replicate in. They don't care if you are genetically a male or a female. They will still infect you. So, let's think about HPV. If HPV is a sexually transmitted disease, that means heterosexual women who are infected can still give it to the men that they have sex with. The virus isn't just going to chill out in the woman's body and be like "heeyyy that's a male body, there's no cervix, I'm just going to stay here". It's going to spread. The virus does cause other cancers. In fact, the virus causes cancers of the vulva, vagina, penis, anus, and the back of the throat[1]. Men are still capable of developing penile, anal and oropharyngeal cancers even if they don't have cervixes! (Oropharyngeal, by the way, is the scientific way of saying throat).

The second vaccine that was available is known as "Gardasil". This vaccine protects against four types of HPV. Specifically, it protects against types 6, 11, 16, and 18. This vaccine requires 3 doses which means that it takes a while to get fully vaccinated. It takes a total of 6 months to get the full set. In all honesty, it seems like a lot of work. However, these vaccines are recommended for young girls and boys starting at the ages of 11 and 12[1]. Many parents are opposed to it because they don't like the idea of their children having sex especially at such a young way.

However, in a way, it's a good thing to get the vaccine that early. The children get the protection before they become sexually active. Their bodies have enough time to create a response and they are capable of engaging in sexual activity when they are ready. On the flip side, imagine getting the vaccine at a much later date, like say when you're 19. You would have to wait six months before you could start becoming sexually active. Like, seriously, what if you had to wait that long? In my opinion, that would be a major bummer. Another point about getting the vaccine early is that the vaccine is also recommended for females from 13 to 26 years of age because that is when the vaccine is most effective[1]. For men, it is recommended from 13 to 21 years of age[1]. There are also recommendations of before and after those ages in case a person wants those series.

One country that has an amazingly effective HPV vaccination program is Australia. In Australia, the vaccine is listed in their immunization program. Schools offer the HPV vaccine for free to both girls and boys from the ages of 12 and 13[21]. Because of this program, Australia is getting very close to eliminating cervical cancer? How? 99.9% of the cervical cancers are caused by STDs, specifically, HPV[1]. By vaccinating children from a young age and by vaccinating girls and boys, the country is getting very close to eliminating the disease. This information, by the way, has been published as of March 2018. For all I know, the country may have successfully eliminated the disease by the time I finish writing this book.

From 2005 to 2015, HPV dropped from 22.7% to 1.1% for Australia women between the ages of 18 and 24[22]. Their immunization rates have also helped make it less likely for young people to come in contact with the virus. In my opinion, Australia has set a really great example. Offering the vaccine for free for children starting at the age of 12 and 13 for both boys and girls ensures that everyone is capable of receiving this health care[21]. The country also offers two doses for free for people who are outside the age range but are under 19[21]. The government is making sure that each child has the opportunity to be protected against a cancer. In contrast, the vaccine can cost around $450 for the entire series[22]. There are also many parents who opt out and the vaccine is mostly still targeted toward just girls. If Australia is capable of eliminating a virus that causes cancer, most developed countries should follow their example. If we have the power to get rid of a cancer, why aren't we doing that?

Onto more advice that may not be applicable to every college student. If you go to a small school or a medium sized school, be careful of who you have sex with. I would highly suggest you try to avoid sleeping with people in the same major or programs as you. Why you might ask? Let's think about it. Imagine a one-night stand with some random person in your major during your freshman year. You might have a great night but you don't really want to be with that person. You could be a jerk and ghost that person. You may even end up in a relationship with that person. Whatever it was, it was just a little college experience you got in your freshman year. Now, let's fast-forward to junior year. Your classes are more major specific and they're much smaller. The next thing you know, that person you slept with once is now your lab partner for the entire semester and they hate you. Yeah, that's no fun. Imagine if you gave them a STD. (Yikes!) That being said, it's only advice and a hypothetical situation that is unlikely to happen. I am not telling you what to do. It's just something to keep in mind.

Generally speaking, the CDC recommends that people do not partake in unsafe sex and try to main healthy, monogamous relationship. Their advice is pretty sound and certainly makes sense as to how it can decrease the amount of disease. But again, it is up to you to determine what types of sexual activity you do and do not partake in. Another piece of advice is abstinence. Abstinence does work to protect against pregnancy and STDs. In this context, abstinence means no sexual activity at all. For some people, that's an unrealistic and undesirable option. For others, it works. It all depends on you.

Now, in the worst-case scenario that you do end up with a STD, remember it is not the end of the world. You live in a time where people can be very supportive. There are more advances in modern medicine. Some diseases are going to be more difficult than others but you can get help. The first step is getting diagnosed. If you think that something is wrong with your health after a sexual encounter. Get a professional medical opinion as soon as you can. The following is a link to the CDC website that can help you find a location that can test you for STDs: https://gettested.cdc.gov/.

If you end up contracting a STD that requires treatment, you could also help your partner get treatment. There is a program known as EPT. EPT stands for "Expedited Partner Therapy"[5]. This program is basically a method of getting treatment for a sexual partner without the process of going through a clinical visit. The clinicians prescribing the medications give sufficient instruction for the prescriptions so that the patients know what to do[5]. The program was created in an attempt to control the spread of STDs as well as to provide treatment for people[6].

As mentioned before, treatment for diseases like gonorrhea and chlamydia are important for females as they can cause infertility when left untreated[6]. Those are a few reasons why this program was created. In the map below, the states with legislature for EPT are marked. If you realize you may have contracted a disease, you could certainly ask your health care provider about this program to help out your partner.

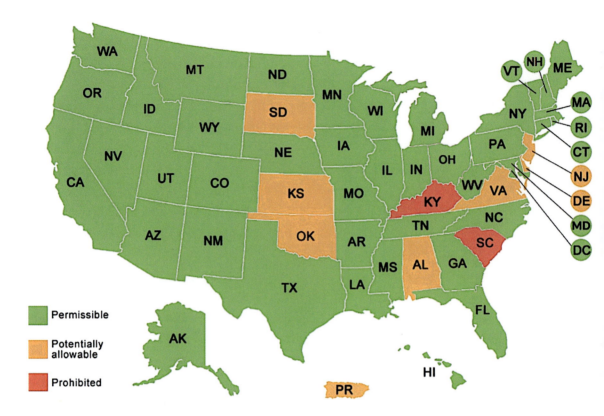

Figure 1. Map of states in the United States and their legal statuses of EPT programs as of 2017[5]

The main point of this chapter: stay safe and make smart decisions. I would highly suggest preparing yourself much in advance since you're definitely not going to care about all these little details in the heat of the moment. College students are notorious for being under the influence of alcohol and other drugs and partaking in risky behaviors. Unsafe sex, remember, is a risky behavior. You can get a lifelong disease by being unsafe!

Be responsible. If not, do everyone a favor, don't have sex. (Yes, that is brutal advice, but your actions have consequences. Don't learn it that the hard way.)

Chapter 6: How to Process Information

Information. It's everywhere. We are incredibly lucky to live in a time where most people have smartphones and can easily fact check or search for information. However, there is a lot of information, like maybe too much? Have you ever stopped to look through all the pages in your Google search? Probably not, we usually gravitate toward the first page and maybe the second page if Google couldn't give us exactly what we wanted. With this awesome power to rapidly find information, there comes a small problem. How do we know what to trust?

As a college student, you are going to have many assignments that require ample research. You are going to have to do some reading and you are going to learn lots of information. However, what information is "good" information and what information is "bad"? Back to our quick little Google search, there is a whole lot of nonsense in the world. How exactly are you going to know what information is trustworthy? What if everything seems trustworthy?

I'll be honest. It's difficult. I have sat in many classes where my professors have asked librarians to come in and explain the different types of sources in the world. I have had to read documents on which types of articles I should be reading. My professors have outlined the differences between popular articles and scholarly articles. Even before high school, I have been taught multiple times to find reliable sources. Clearly, there are many people who don't know how to do that if all these teachers and professors are spending time on it? Right? Yep. People do not use reliable resources all the time. You are going to have fellow classmates who still do not know how to find reliable information (scary when you think about group projects) and classmates who do not know how to cite information properly.

This chapter is not going to go into details regarding academic research, I'll leave that to your professors since it varies slightly from profession to profession. Regardless of whether you are doing scientific research or English research, it's important to learn how to do it right. Trust me. Instead, this chapter is going to give you a quick tutorial on how you can determine the reliability of medical sources. You may even find yourself explaining this process to a friend or family member.

When looking at online resources, consider four aspects of the source before you decide to consume the knowledge. These four aspects are transparency, presentation, commercialization, and funding[7]. There are other aspects that could also be considered as well, but these are the four that I am going to focus on.

Transparency

Does this website tell you who is in charge? Can you find contact information? Does this website list sources? Can you tell who and where this information is from? Transparency is extremely important for websites that present medical information. If it is not clear who is giving you the information, you may want to reconsider your source.

Think about it this way. If you're in a relationship with someone, you want that person to be honest with you. You would hope they aren't hiding anything from you. It's transparent because you can see everything clearly and not worry. This same concept should be applied to where information, especially medical information, is coming from. When you look at medical information, you probably want to know who is telling you the information. What is in their background in medicine/science? Are they complete and thorough in the information?

Many websites provide contact information. There is often a page that lists people and their credentials. Always, and I mean always, search for who is giving you the information. If there is page that lists contact information, search that person up. Find out where they studied. Look for their specialties. Check out the credentials. There are some people who lie. Yes, there are adults who lie on their resumes and lie about their expertise. Don't fall victim to that. Check where they studied and see if you can confirm it. You would be surprised but some people will lie about this information. There are also some people who are very good at sounding, looking and behaving professional. There is a difference between sounding professional and being professional. Just because someone has a big and fancy title doesn't necessarily mean they are 100% reliable. Look it up. If the website is run by a group or organization, you should be able to find basic information about them such as their goals or mission. Typically, the "about us" link can help you find as much information as you can. The main point, find out who is providing the information on the website. *make sure they're not lying*

Presentation

Does the website look professional? If your answer is no, you definitely shouldn't trust it for information. Maybe look around for a laugh or two because it could be good for entertainment purposes. Certainly, don't count it as a reliable source. If yes, the website does look professional, then look at the headlines[7]. One way to determine if a website is reliable is by reading the headlines and titles. The headlines from scientific sources should avoid bias. They should also avoid emotionally charged language[7]. They should typically avoid anything that seems "miraculous" or too good to be true. For instance, the website shouldn't have headlines such as "Extreme Life Extension and the Search for Immortality" (which by the way was a headline that was found on mercola.com). The website should also be easy to navigate. If it is difficult to find certain information or just click around, that may be a little warning that the website isn't as legitimate as it seems.

Commercialization

Does this website have multiple commercials? Is it trying to sell me something? Are there links to products that claim to improve life? In terms of medical information, you may want to steer clear of a website that has many ads on it. Also, make sure to stay away if there is someone trying to sell a very specific product that claims to have miracle effects. For instance, if the website is telling you to buy a supplemental pill that claims to cure cancer, avoid that website. If it was as simple as a pill, then cancer wouldn't be such a large issue. Also, wouldn't it be weird if only one person was claiming to have the cure? Wouldn't pharmaceutical companies be trying to profit from these cures as well? It's just a little weird and sketchy when these miracle products are all over the website.

For the most part, reliable medical sites should not be asking you to buy products. They should be receiving enough funding. Sometimes they ask for donations, but they will be very clear about where the money is going. For example, the Immunization Action Coalition is a nonprofit organization that focuses on providing accurate vaccine information. Their website has a "Make a Donation" tab. It takes you to a page that explains their goals and purposes before you decide to make a donation. Just like any other website, think for a while before spending any of your money. If you are looking at website, it shouldn't have so many ads that it looks like it's going to give your computer a virus. + it shouldn't be selling you stuff

Funding

Who is funding this website? Every website has to have an owner and every website has to have some source of financial support. It's very easy to make your own website and maintain it. Honestly, anyone with a stable income and a credit card can run a website and everyone has access to it. Most major organizations provide the information on their websites. There is just a little digging involved. For instance, on the American Association of Pediatrics, their financial reports can be found. In a way, funding and transparency can go hand in hand.

Consider who is funding the website in terms of any personal interests or conflicts. For instance, if a company is funding a website, they will want to present information that would help benefit their company. For instance, let's imagine there is a brand new and very popular fitness website. This website is giving all sorts of information that seems fairly valid. However, they post about how sugary sports drinks are absolutely necessary to obtain the summer body that everyone wants. You do some research and you find out a soda company funds the website. That makes sense now. It is in the financial interest of the soda company to sell sugary drinks to make money. They need people to buy their products so they are not going to provide or promote information that could hurt their business. In the same way, there have been people against vaccines who have personal interests that drive them to make false claims about vaccines. They could be paid. They could have their own products they are trying to sell. Basically, conflicts of interests are very important to consider when it comes to funding and most funding should be easy to identify.

Another important aspect of doing any research is cross-referencing. Try to obtain your information from a variety of sources. Biases are prevalent everywhere in the world.

As a college student, you should definitely learn how to decide when people are biased toward one perspective. However, sometimes that is difficult to figure out especially when the perspective they are reporting is the same as your perspective. Vary your sources so you can get the full picture and see what other perspectives also exist. Often times, one side of the story is not enough to fully understand a report or topic. In terms of medical advice, sometimes you go to multiple doctors for a medical opinion. You should do the same when it comes to controversial information. Find multiple sources and compare the information. for controversial topics

As mentioned, cross-referencing is important. Cross-referencing is essentially checking to find the same information from different sources. If these sources give the same consensus on a topic, it could be safe to say that information is reliable. However, you could also be cross-referencing using unreliable sources. Some unreliable websites link to other websites that also provide misinformation. In this scenario, check to see if these websites are reliable. If a seemingly reliable website links to a very unreliable website with lots of commercials, there may be a problem. A reliable website should link to other reliable websites. Finding reliable sources is very possible but it does require some work sometimes.

On another note, remember that you shouldn't be getting all your information from your favorite celebrity. Depending on the celebrity, always take into consideration their expertise. If your celebrity is a model, dispensing medical advice, when she has no medical training, don't listen to that medical advice! Instead find a medical professional who has been trained properly and knows their information. Try to consider that their beliefs may not be fact. As mentioned, there are many people who broadcast their beliefs. Sometimes, celebrities don't even broadcast their beliefs. They may endorse products or services that they disagree with. In those cases, companies may be providing them with a solid amount of money for the celebrity endorsement.

Now, I'm going to focus more on scientific journals. There are many of them out in the world. There are so many scholarly, peer-reviewed journals. Many universities and college libraries try to give their students access to databases full of these peer-reviewed journals. Definitely utilize those resources if your university provides them. It will certainly help you find more reliable information than a simple Google search. With that being said, Google searches can also help with finding trustworthy and scholarly articles from journals. I also mentioned the word "peer-review".

What exactly does that mean? It means that the journal was read and reviewed by another expert that does not work for the journal. This scientist has to look over the study to ensure that it fits criteria for the journal. They also check for quality and importance of the materials that they are sent to review. Peer-review is a way to ensure that there is are proper scientific practices being performed and data presentation. The reviewer must be an expert in the field in which the journal specializes to ensure that the study is being reviewed for the right information[1].

Among the sea of trustworthy journals, there are so many imposters. One of the most important lessons I learned in my research class was that predatory journals exist. Yes, predatory journals. These are often journals that look very official and send researchers lots of emails asking them for submissions. These journals look and act very official. Many of them also ask you to pay them money in order to get your paper published. In the scientific community, these journals are a huge pain. The sad part is that some young scientists probably don't know about them. They get this incredibly prestigious looking journal that is emailing them about their research. However, it is probably just someone trying to scam them out of their money. There are also scientists who submit to these journals just so they can claim that they are published. These journals are often not reviewed and have no actual value to them. Don't believe me? I suggest you read the following journal. It's very enlightening.

Get me off Your Fucking Mailing List

David Mazières and Eddie Kohler
New York University
University of California, Los Angeles
http://www.mailavenger.org/

Abstract

Get me off your fucking mailing list. Get me off your fucking mailing list. Get me off your fucking mailing list. Get me off your fucking mailing list. Get me off your fucking mailing list. Get me off your fucking mailing list. Get me off your fucking mailing list. Get me off your fucking mailing list. Get me off your fucking mailing list. Get me off your fucking mailing list. Get me off your fucking mailing list. Get me off your fucking mailing list. Get me off your fucking mailing list. Get me off your fucking mailing list.

1 Introduction

Get me off your fucking mailing list. Get me off your fucking mailing list. Get me off your fucking mailing list. Get me off your fucking mailing list. Get me off your fucking mailing list. Get me off your fucking mailing list. Get me off your fucking mailing list. Get me off your fucking mailing list. Get me off your fucking mailing list. Get me off your fucking mailing list. Get me off your fucking mailing list. Get me off your fucking mailing list. Get me off your fucking mailing list. Get me off your fucking mailing list. Get me off your fucking mailing list. Get me off your fucking mailing list. Get me off your fucking mailing list.

Get me off your fucking mailing list. Get me off your fucking mailing list. Get me off your fucking mailing list. Get me off your fucking mailing list. Get me off your fucking mailing list. Get me off your fucking mailing list. Get me off your fucking mailing list. Get me off your fucking mailing list. Get me off your fucking mailing list. Get me off your fucking mailing list. Get me off your fucking mailing list. Get me off your fucking mailing list. Get me off your fucking mailing list. Get me off your fucking mailing list.

Get me off your fucking mailing list. Get me off your fucking mailing list. Get me off your fucking

Figure 1. Page from a "Get me off Your Fucking Mail List" [2]

You're probably thinking, "there is no way that is real." Let me tell you, it is indeed very real. In my research class, my professor showed us this very document to demonstrate how anyone can get published. Many scientists get bombarded with emails from these predatory journals. Some of them get so fed up, they decide to actually submit jokes to prove how anything can be published. As you can see, the UCLA researchers in the "Get me Off Your Fucking Mailing List" study, just copied and pasted the same phrase multiple times. The article was not published as the researchers did not want to pay $150 to publish it[9].

Other scientists have published fake studies to also demonstrate how easy it is for fake science to be spread to the public. For instance, there was this study that was going around about how chocolate can actually help people lose weight. This article was fairly popular. Why shouldn't it be? Most people love chocolate and it would be awesome if it could help with weight loss. The journal article was published by Dr. John Bohannon and his colleagues,
Their goal for their study was to show how easy it is for bad science to get published.

The study was titled "Chocolate with high Cocoa content as a weight-loss accelerator"[3]. The authors are listed as Johannes Bohannon, Diana Koch, Peter Homm, and Alexander Direhaus. These authors all worked together and performed an actual study and submitted their real findings. This study had participants between the ages of 19 and 67[4]. They took the participants and put them into three groups. One group was put on a low-carb diet. Another group was put on that low-carb diet but were also given a daily serving of chocolate that was 81% cocoa[4]. The final group weren't given a specific diet, they were allowed to eat whatever they pleased. The participants were followed for three weeks.

For the overall study, the researchers looked at many different variables. They looked at weight, cholesterol, sodium, blood protein levels, sleep-quality, and well-being. They looked at other variables as well and it totaled to about 18 different measurements[2]. The overall study found that the participants in the low-carb chocolate group experienced 10% more weight loss than just the low-carb diet[4]. Their results were real, so what's the catch?

Here's the catch: the study had a very small number of people and many variables that they were considering. According to Dr. Bohannon in his article about their study, a researcher can easily produce significant results if the total number of participants is very small. The researcher is also able to get some sort of significant result if the he looks at many variables. The more variables, the more likely something has to be significant[2]. Basically, the more variables that are looked at increases the likelihood that something would be statistically significant.

What does it mean if something is statistically significant? It means that in a T-test (this is one method of statistical analysis), that the results had a small p value. Usually the p value cut-off is 0.05. This value indicates that there is a 5% chance that the data may get a random fluctuation. According to Dr. Bohannon, the chocolate study had a 60% chance of something resulting in a statistically significant result (so a result less than 0.05). This tactic is apparently called "p-hacking" which is basically creating a study so that you can purposefully get results that are less than 0.05. I think that it's sort of like scientific cheating. However, there are scientists who do it without realizing and these scientists aren't lying about their results. That usually results in scientists repeating their experiments until they get the results that they want. They're basically just doing something over and over again until they get it to "work" in their favor[2].

This study also had other issues that many people didn't consider. For instance, Dr. Bohannon mentioned how none of the reporters who contacted him asked about how many participants were in his study[2]. Just to point this out, when I first read his study, I looked around everywhere for how many people he had in his study. I couldn't find it anywhere which I thought was rather odd. Upon finding his article explaining this study, I discovered there were only 15 people in the study[2]. Let me just say that is a tiny study. The introduction made it sound like they had a large number of people as their age range was 19 to 67. Clearly, that was not the case.

His article also pointed out that journals are getting better about which studies they accept. Many journals won't accept studies with less than 30 participants[2]. The reason why is that small studies don't have enough people. There should be large numbers of people whose ages and genders balance out in all the different variable groups. A large number of participants helps avoid confounding variables from having too much of an effect.

For instance, in this study, Dr. Bohannon mentioned that a woman's weight can fluctuate five pounds during her menstrual cycle. This study did not take this into consideration and failed to control this variable. This variable would be very important for their study as the five pounds is much greater than the weight difference between the two groups in their results[2].

Basically, large numbers provide a method of control so that data provide a more accurate depiction of the results. Another important change that Dr. Bohannon mentioned regarding journals is that they are trying to phase out of using p values as the main indicator of significant results. He says that journals are doing this so that scientists are more likely to practice and conduct correct and proper scientific behavior.

This study was submitted to a number of predatory journals. The researchers chose the International Archives of Medicine. They paid 600 euros so that this study could be published[2]. Once it was published, the media ate it up. I mean, like, they literally ate it up. Why wouldn't they? Chocolate for weight loss? That would be awesome. This study was everywhere during 2015. The best part was Dr. Bohannon literally got advice from his friend who works in public relations and created the perfect story for journalists to eat up. They even had some freelance artists create some video clips for their weight loss study. The plan certainly worked. They had articles from the *Daily Star,* the *Irish*

Examiner, Times of India and the German and Indian sites of the Huffington Post[2]. This study really got some attention. I think the best part is that really does show how easy unreliable science can become incredibly popular.

However, among the crowd of scientists who want to publish real and reliable science to prevail, there are many scientists who are focused on publishing and receiving credit. Some scientists don't care if they conduct their research ethically or if their results are even accurate. There are many scientists who are only focused on the fame and the money. There are also scientists who are just very desperate for publication because they need to build their resumes. It's sad to admit but not every scientist, or person, has pure intentions. Money and prestige are just two motivators that cause corruption. This corruption can lead to false data and misinformation that can harm many lives.

Scientific studies are also not very easy to read. They can be full of very difficult jargon and it's understandable as to why some people just don't read the studies. It can be very hard, especially if you're not trained or interested in science. Overall, I think it's important to be wary of scientific studies especially when the media is screaming about miraculous or maybe even terrifying results.

Since this book is on vaccines, I've decided to provide some reliable and unreliable websites you can visit to see the differences yourself. I learned about many of these websites from *Your Baby's Best Shot: Why Vaccines are Safe and Save Lives*. This book is written for parents who are curious about vaccines. They compiled websites that provide accurate vaccine information as well as websites that perpetuate vaccine misinformation. Below are the reliable websites and following that list are the unreliable websites. The links are provided so you can look compare and contrast them yourselves. In my opinion, the anti-vaccine websites are slightly concerning and very laughable. You may disagree but I still suggest clicking around to see the nonsense for yourself. Some of it is very well-done and can easily deter an unaware viewer into the wrong direction.

Reliable Websites with Vaccine Information
The American Academy of Pediatrics: https://www.aap.org/en-us/Pages/Default.aspx

The American Academy of Pediatrics is an organization of 66,000 pediatricians. I don't know about you, but that's a lot of doctors specialized in taking care of children. Like think about it, that many professional and trained people are "committed to the optimal physical, mental, and social health and well-being for all infants, children, adolescents, and young adults"[10]. Just to make this clear, that statement is found word for word on the AAP website on their "About the AAP" page. When you go to this page, there is also a video used a method to explain the AAP. Below the video, there are subcategories of information regarding the AAP. There is a category for facts about the organization.

One category for committees, councils, and sections of the AAP. The best part is that when you click the section labeled "AAP Facts" it takes you to another page that has more subheadings. The very last subheading is a link to all their financial information demonstrates a significant amount of transparency. There is also a page for contact information which directs you to many other resources along with the contact information. The website is also devoid of any commercialization. There is also a link to how they are funded. In terms of any form of product selling, the AAP has the "shopAAP" link which sells some of their products. However, there isn't just one doctor claiming that their book is to answer to all the questions a parent could have. Overall, I think this website is certainly professional, informational and reliable on many topics besides vaccines.

The Centers for Disease Control: https://www.cdc.gov/

The Centers for Disease Control is a federal public health agency for the United States. The website doesn't have any commercialization. The website is pretty simple to navigate. On this page, the CDC explains how they can be linked. For instance, their short explanation is the following, "Short: CDC.gov is your online source for credible health information and is the official Web site of the Centers for Disease Control and Prevention (CDC)". It's very short and sweet and direct. The long version of their description is the following:

> Long: CDC.gov is your online source for credible health information and is the official Web site of the Centers for Disease Control and Prevention (CDC). CDC is committed to achieving true improvements in people's health. CDC applies research and findings to improve people's daily lives and responds to health emergencies—something that distinguishes CDC from its peer agencies. Working with states and other partners, CDC provides a system of health surveillance to monitor and prevent disease outbreaks (including bioterrorism), implement disease prevention strategies, and maintain national health statistics. CDC also guards against international disease transmission, with personnel stationed in more than 25 foreign countries.[11]

At the very bottom of the "About Us" page, the website has a "Page last reviewed" and a "Page last updated" which lets you know how old the information could potentially be. Underneath those dates, there is also a link that says "Page maintained by: Office of the Associate Director for Communication, Division of Public Affairs" which lets you know who is in charge of that page. The website also provides a funding link at the very bottom of their homepage.

The CDC is one of the United States' leading public health agencies. They provide many resources and reliable information. For instance, most of this book is written using information from their book *Epidemiology and prevention of vaccine-preventable diseases*. They try to provide information in a manner that most people are capable of reading and understanding. Overall, I would say that the CDC is definitely a reliable and useful resource for many different topics related to health care.

The Immunization Action Coalition: http://www.immunize.org/

This website has been mentioned earlier in this chapter. The website is run by a nonprofit organization that wants to facilitate and provide correct information about vaccines. They want to make sure people are not getting sick from vaccine preventable diseases. The website does ask for donations which is why it was mentioned above. However, looking through the website, one can easily tell it is a reliable source of medical information. The website is professional looking. It has many links at the very bottom of the page that makes navigation easy. The purpose of the group is very clear. There are no insane advertisements for strange pills. No one is endorsing their own books. There are some products that are up for sale. These products include a DVD on immunizations, a laminated vaccine schedule and record cards.

The website also cites other websites such as the WHO, CDC, and ACIP. In fact, the IAC's mission statement mentions that they have worked closely with CDC for at least two decades to educate health care professionals. Upon further observation, this website has unbiased headings. The headings also provide information without any false promises or miracles. For anyone looking for more information on vaccines, this website is certainly a useful find. I personally find that it sounds very fancy, like how often do people refer to themselves as a "coalition"? Probably more than I realize, but I still think it's pretty fancy.

The Vaccine Education Center at the Children's Hospital of Philadelphia:
http://www.chop.edu/centers-programs/vaccine-education-center

This website was made by the Children's Hospital of Philadelphia. This hospital was the United States' first pediatric hospital. It has been a center of research and development for many health initiatives including vaccines. The Vaccine Education Center was created to educate people about vaccines and provide accurate and updated information. On the website, there are many links to different topics related to vaccines. There are no advertisements. There is a contact the VEC link on the website. This website also provides more specific information regarding the VEC team. This link is pretty impressive because it takes you to the Vaccine Education Center team. Each person on the team has a link that takes you to more information about them. Some of these team members have their photos and others do not. Each team member has a link There is information regarding all of their credentials. For instance, Dr. Paul Offit has all his information on his page. His page gives his education and training, where he currently works, any academic titles, and so much more information regarding his credentials. This website is very simple and easy to navigate. Overall, it is definitely a reliable and trustworthy source.

Unreliable Websites with Vaccine (mis)Information
Mercola.com: https://www.mercola.com/

Dr. Mercola is a doctor from Illinois. His website's main purpose is to provide information about natural health[7]. Yes, natural health. As of 2018, there are many people who are looking around for "natural" remedies and equate "natural" to healthier. There are a few issues with this craze but that isn't the purpose of this book. I will go over a related and very common related misconception.

Back to Dr. Mercola, he is incredibly popular and has many subscribers and followers on both his Twitter and Facebook accounts. His website is all about natural health remedies. There are many different links but is rather difficult to navigate. There are also many different advertisements at the bottom of his website. If you look through his website, there are many topics that he covers besides vaccines. Interestingly enough, when trying to go through all the videos he has on vaccines, the viewer cannot go past the first page of videos. I can't really figure out why it's set up like that. His website is not the most professional website either. Especially when compared to the CDC and CHOP's Vaccine Education Center page.

The website has a toll-free number that someone could use to call. I'm not really sure who this phone number takes you to but it exists. This website also sends you to Dr. Mercola's shop that sells "Dr. Mercola Premium Products". I don't know about you but this page is definitely a red flag to me. There are so many supplements that require you to pay a pretty penny to obtain these products (but don't worry, I think there's free shipping for some products?). The website sells stuff like krill oil, fermented black garlic pills, and 100% Grass Fed Frozen Beef Marrow Bones[12]. Just so you know, as I am writing this book, the beef marrow bones currently have free shipping. Basically, this website is full of questionable information and products and there are definitely people who whole-heartedly believe in Dr. Mercola. I mean, he's a doctor, we can trust him? (I am really hoping your answer was no).

ThinkTwice: http://thinktwice.com/

This website is probably one of the less professional looking websites. I'm not entirely sure who is in charge or the website or who runs it. There is an "About Us" link which provides some clear information. The page discusses *New Atlantean Press* and how it was established to publish holistic books. It continues by discussing that the ThintkTwice Global Vaccine Institute was created in 1996 to give parents information about vaccines so they can make more informed information. When reading the page further, there is link that says "DISCLAIMER". Upon clicking this link, the following disclaimer in the figure below shows up.

> **Disclaimer**
> - The information contained within the Thinktwice Global Vaccine Institute website is for educational and informational purposes only, and is not to be construed as medical advice. Licensed health practitioners are available for this purpose.
> - The Thinktwice Global Vaccine Institute has endeavored to provide accurate and credible information. However, errors can occur. Therefore, readers are urged to verify all of the data on this website.
> - Some of the information presented on the Thinktwice Global Vaccine Institute website may conflict with data presented elsewhere. Therefore, readers are encouraged to remain circumspect and use discretion when interpreting contradictory, complex or confusing concepts.
> - The Thinktwice Global Vaccine Institute is not endorsed by pharmaceutical companies, the American Academy of Pediatrics, the FDA, CDC or any other federal, state or "official" organization. For official information about vaccines, contact vaccine manufacturers, the FDA, CDC or World Health Organization.
> - Vaccine recommendations change rapidly. Immunization schedules are periodically revised. Therefore, the FDA and CDC -- not the Thinktwice Global Vaccine Institute -- should be consulted for the most up-to-date information regarding who should or should not receive vaccines, at what ages, and the number of doses.
> - The Thinktwice Global Vaccine Institute does not recommend for or against vaccines. Parents and other concerned people must make this decision on their own. Because the data on this website tends to implicate vaccines (find fault with them), readers are advised to balance the data presented here with data presented by "official" sources of vaccine information, including pharmaceutical companies, the FDA, CDC and World Health Organization.
> - The decision regarding whether or not to vaccinate is a personal one. The authors of the Thinktwice Global Vaccine Institute website are neither health practitioners nor legal advisors, and make no claims in this regard. Therefore, none of the information on this website should be construed as medical or legal advice. No one associated with this website recommends for or against vaccines. If you have questions regarding any of the information on this website, research immunizations to a greater degree so that you can make wise and informed decisions.

Figure 2. Disclaimer from ThinkTwice.com[8]

    I find this disclaimer very important. It literally says that the information is for educational purpose but it can't be used as medical advice. The website also says that the FDA and the CDC should be consulted for vaccine schedules. However, clicking around the website can show any viewer how they are still giving false information. How many people do you think even read the disclaimer?

    In an attempt to try to find contact information, I clicked on the "Email Us" link which was fairly easy to find. However, I'm not really sure who I'm contacting but I managed to find an email address. As I explored this website some more, I found other interesting pages. There is a page on vaccine laws: http://thinktwice.com/laws.htm. This page looks like a sample question and answer format. They clearly say "Sample Letter" next to some of the questions but this example makes it seem as if there are people who are actually asking these questions. I scrolled through and picked some questions that I thought were interesting. For instance, the website in figure 3 cites an unreliable source, the NVIC. The NVIC is an unreliable source which will be discussed later in this chapter. How could someone trust a website that is citing another unreliable source?

2. Are vaccines mandatory for my children to get into a public daycare, school, or college?

Response:
In most states, vaccines are NOT required to enroll in a public daycare, school or college. Most states offer a philosophical or religious exemption. Acquire a copy of the vaccine laws of your state to learn about your rights. Then write and submit an exemption. (Some states provide their own exemption form.) You can research the laws on your own or use the map below provided by the National Vaccine Information Center.

On the map below, click on the state that you are interested in to learn more about that state's vaccine exemption laws.

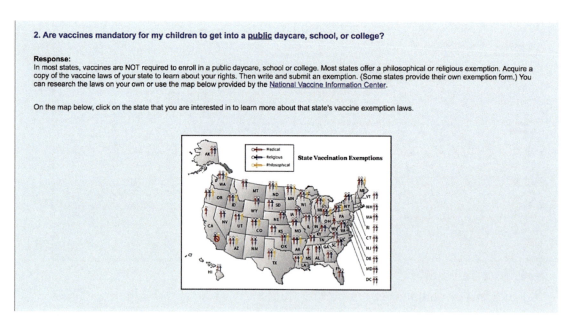

Figure 3. Sample Question and Answer from ThinkTwice.com[8]

In figure 4, there is a question about vaccines and international travel. I found this question interesting because the website is presenting the idea that hepatitis A "is not that bad". From an earlier chapter, we know that's not the case. A person viewing this website could read that and think that the sample letter must be right since it's written online. Sometimes, people are just quickly skimming and they don't focus on what the writing actually says. In those cases, a viewer could get the wrong information and harm themselves as well as those around them.

5. I am a U.S. citizen and plan to travel to a foreign country. Are vaccines mandatory for me and my family?

Response:
Vaccines are rarely required for travel from the United States to foreign destinations. They may be recommended but are rarely required, despite what some pushy and misinformed health authorities may tell you. Some vaccines, such as the yellow fever shot, may be required when traveling to rural regions of Africa or South America during seasons when yellow fever infection is officially reported. Check the CDC's travel website for more information.

Sample Letter:
I'm about to go abroad to South America. I don't want to take the recommended vaccines because I really believe in my body. Yellow fever, however, is from a mosquito and some people die from it. Hepatitis A is not that bad, if I'm informed. Anyway, what do you think about those travel vaccines? Are they really just moneymakers for corporations or are travel vaccines different than vaccines for children?

All vaccines pose risks that must be weighed against their purported benefits. Travel vaccines can harm adults just as childhood vaccines can harm children. Of course, some people are harmed from the diseases, so you must do your research. To help with your research, the Vaccine Safety Manual has a chapter wholly devoted to travel vaccines, including vaccines for yellow fever, typhoid fever, cholera, japanese encephalitis, and more.

Figure 4. Question regarding travel from ThinkTwice.com[8]

Another important point is that this page uses anecdotes to create a stronger impact on their readers. What does that mean? Typically, people are more likely to remember personal stories (anecdotes). These anecdotes are often personal and helps a person feel more connected. These stories play on emotions and are much easier for most people to remember. This website basically uses the emotional response to enforce their point of view. In fact, the "Personal Stories" tab is evidence that the website relies on anecdotes. Based on my exploration, I don't think it's very accurate. There seems to be a strong reliance on emotion rather than science. I wouldn't consider this source useful or trustworthy.

Whale.to: http://whale.to/

This website is probably the least professional looking website out of all of the ones listed. I honestly can't even figure out the purpose of this website. For instance, why is it called "Whale"? Since this website looks pretty sketchy, it already seems like it can't be considered a reliable source. There doesn't look like there is overt commercialization. There is a link for the history behind the website. On the page, there is a disclaimer. There is also explanation for the name "Whale".

The website is basically run by a man, John Scudamore, who just complies information that he thinks is valid. Reading this page gives you what can only be an autobiography of a man who believes in the Auschwitz Hoax and Cancer Genocide. Basically, this is the perfect example of how anyone can own a website. According to the *Your Baby's Best Shot: Why Vaccines are Safe and Save Lives,* Scudamore is an English pig farmer. Yes, a pig farmer is spreading medical information and some people may actually believe him. I don't know if his website is very popular but it exists and anyone can happen upon this page.

National Vaccine Information Center: https://www.nvic.org/

Now, this website. If you click on it, you will notice that this website is very professional looking. It looks like the information is reliable. For an unsuspecting person, this website can and will be very misleading. The name of the website, "National Vaccine Information Center," also sounds convincingly official to me. It says that the website is run entirely by donations. The headings look like they are mostly unbiased. There is one video on there currently that "Baylor's Doc Hotez Bullies Parents of Vaccine Injured Children" which is a link to a video by Barbara Loe Fischer[6]. The title of the video is emotionally charged as it does attack Dr. Hotez which indicates that this website is slightly unreliable. In all honesty, this website seems fairly normal. However, it states that it is partners with Mercola.com which to me is a big red flag.

The most concerning part about this website is that it has an "International Memorial for Vaccine Victims". This page is about honoring the lives of people who have been killed by vaccines. The page takes you to a search engine to find specific people are no longer alive. I have a few questions. What about all the people who have died from the diseases that these vaccines prevent? Where are those people's names? Where are the names of all the children who die because of diseases like measles? What about all the children who died of polio? What about all the deaths of people dying of hepatitis B? Is this memorial a fair depiction of vaccines?

As you can see, some websites are fairly easy to navigate. Some websites are very clearly unreliable. The websites can look very professional or very unprofessional. Facts are powerful. Data is powerful. Sound science is powerful. Ask people where they're getting their information. Most of the time, I fall victim to this too, people can't cite their sources. Backing yourself and your argument with evidence is very important. Learn to do that properly and effectively. Learn to do that with valid information. Also learn to be receptive and willing to listen in case your information is wrong.

I hope by now, you know you can't trust everything that you read. If there is ever a time when you are questioning reliability and validity, search deeper. Look for other sources to cross-reference. With that being said, I would obviously say I'm pretty reliable. However, you know where to look to double-check to make sure. (Hint: check the references at the end of this book).

Chapter 7: Myths

In the first chapter, I mentioned that you're going to meet many people in the world with different beliefs than you. You're going to meet many people who are going to disagree with you and many people who agree with you. Remember, opinions are not facts. The sky is blue. That is a fact. Blue is an ugly color. That statement is not a fact, that is an opinion (I, by the way, love the color blue and think it's beautiful).

For some reason, many people have this belief that their opinions are facts and that they're always right. Some of these people may be very vocal about their opinions and they're going to sound very persuasive. They may try a variety of methods to force their opinion on you. For instance, they may aggressively say you're wrong and attack your personality (even though they just met you?). The bottom line is that you are going to encounter so many different opinions. Many of these opinions may be based on myths.

Personally, I think that hardest part is not having enough information. For that reason, I want to arm you with the correct information regarding vaccines. That way, when you meet someone who has misinformation, you can go into battle and fight this person to the death! In reality, I would hope you would gently talk to the person and explain to them why they are wrong. (that, by the way, may be much easier said than actually done…)

When it comes to vaccines, there are so many myths. There is so much misinformation. There are so many books that try to debunk these myths. However, I hope to provide some information that can help anyone debunk these myths when they hear them.

MYTH: *Vaccines give you the disease.*

As we earned earlier, there are many people who claim that the flu shot gave them the flu. In some rare cases, there are people who have severe reactions and medically cannot receive the flu shot. However, most of the vaccines are not going to give you the disease that they are supposed to protect you against. The vaccines contain a safer version of the pathogen. Just a reminder, the influenza viruses in the shot have all been killed or inactivated so that they cannot cause harm. If anything, a person can become sick because they were infected with a different pathogen. That person's body may even be producing an immune response to that vaccine.

With that being said, historically, there have been live oral polio vaccines that infected people with polio. These vaccines were made poorly and were given to people in 1955[2]. This issue is known as the "Cutter Incident"[2]. Essentially, Cutter Laboratories was a company that had produced the live oral polio vaccine. They had made a mistake in producing it and caused 40,000 cases of polio[2]. Of those cases, 200 people were left with different types of paralysis and 10 people were killed[2]. That being said, the United States switched to using just the inactivated polio vaccine in 2000. I know that was at least one man, John Salamone, who worked hard from switching the United States over to the inactivated vaccine after his son had contracted polio from the oral vaccine[5]. From every mistake, there are typically lessons that are learned. For that reason and many other reasons, vaccine safety has been improving. Overall, vaccines are not designed to give people diseases.

MYTH: *Too many vaccines are harmful to your body.*

There is a myth that exists among parents that too many vaccines at once is harmful to the body. This myth is mostly surrounded around the idea that babies get too many vaccines and their immune systems are too fragile to handle all those chemicals[1]. This idea is called "immune overload." Immune overload, my friends, does not exist. The myth is completely false.

Let's discuss babies. Babies develop in the wombs of their mothers. The mother's body protects and houses the fetus until it is born. The womb is sterile and clean. Once the baby leaves the birth canal, it is exposed to countless antigens! There are so many microorganisms around, wouldn't there be immune overload right then and there? The baby encounters all of these antigens all at once and does not experience any form of immune overload.

The concept of immune overload also doesn't make much sense if you think about it in other contexts either. The world is teeming with microorganisms that can cause people to get sick. Just go to a playground and you can see children running around in the dirt and playing on the swings and slides. All of those children just came into contact with all sorts of germs. Wouldn't their bodies be incapable of handling all those antigens?

Vaccines in comparison don't have that many antigens. Each vaccine contains between 1 and 69 antigens[3]. According to the CDC, children receive up to 315 antigens through vaccination by the age of two[3]. In comparison, the smallpox vaccine had 200 antigens in it[4]. All the vaccines that were given in 1980, had around 3200 proteins in it[4]. These vaccines included smallpox, diphtheria, tetanus, pertussis and polio. Fast-forward to 1980, take away smallpox but add measles, mumps, and rubella. In total, there were around 3000 proteins in all of these vaccines[4]. Yes, there are more shots that are given but each shot contains far fewer antigens.

Humans are interesting because we all have the same bodies with many, many differences. The differences in genes allow for some much variability between people. All of us have so differences in our bodies. For instance, some people are more susceptible to addiction to drugs. Some people are more likely to gain weight while others are not. Just like these genetic differences exist, immune system responses can vary between individuals. For instance, I could have two people get the same vaccine. One person is capable of creating 85% of the immune response necessary to be protected against the disease. The other person could only create 60%. For that reason, multiple doses for specific vaccines are recommended. How exactly do we make sure that people have the right amount of protection? Health care professionals can check a person's titer. A titer is a test that is done to determine the levels of antibodies circulating in a person's blood. Titers require a health care professional to draw some blood (probably a few vials). These titers can be performed to determine if a person has enough immunity, if not, they can get a booster shot.

MYTH: *Delaying vaccines is better.* [1]

There are many parents in the world who think that it is their right to determine when their babies and children can receive vaccines. Some of them even think that they can follow an alternative schedule that was created by a man known as Dr. Bob Sears. Dr. Sears has a book that outlines and explains that vaccines aren't to be trusted and that they should be delayed[1].

Delaying vaccines is not helpful and it is definitely not better for people. The idea is that fewer vaccines at once is better for a baby. That idea is far from the truth. The recommendations from the CDC have been set purposefully. These vaccines are given at times so that children are protected at an ideal time.

One issue is that the delayed schedule means there are children who go to schools, go to parks, go to doctor's offices without being vaccinated. These children could contract measles or maybe mumps or maybe the chickenpox and spread these diseases to younger children who have not been vaccinated. Remember, they aren't even vaccinated until 12 months of age. They could also put immunocompromised students at risk.

Unvaccinated children could potentially even put you at risk. Think about it, many college students want to work with children or volunteer their time. If you're working with children, you could be potentially put in contact with unvaccinated children if your titers are low.

In terms of your college life, you may consider delaying the HPV vaccine. As already discussed in an earlier chapter, it takes about 6 months for the entire vaccine series to be completed. As a reminder, the statistics also say that it is better for females to be vaccinated at 13 to 26 years and 13 to 21 for males. So, what do you think? Should people delay vaccines?

MYTH: *Natural Immunity is better.* [1]

There are some people in the world who believe that natural immunity is better than "artificially" acquiring the disease. Take a moment and think about the VPDs that were discussed in an earlier chapter in this book. Do you want to get measles and be immunocompromised for two to three years? How about getting rotavirus multiple times? Or would you rather get Hepatitis B?

No, seriously, think about it. Which diseases do you think you would want to experience naturally? Polio has three strains which means you would have to contract and survive all three types of polio in order to be immune to the disease. Each time you get polio, there's the chance of dying. Rotavirus doesn't ensure full immunity after the first infection. You would need to experience severe diarrhea multiple times in order to gain the immunity necessary to protect yourself from the virus. Each time you are infected with the virus and get the disease, you're again risking the chance of dying.

Why would you want to put yourself at risk of dying multiple times? What about HPV? There are so many different strains and you could potentially get cancer. Imagine that you naturally got the disease and then you would have to fight off the cancer. Wouldn't you rather gain protection without risking the cancer?

It would make sense to gain protection from these diseases without ever actually getting these diseases. There are vaccines readily available that can provide protection. Why should you risk it?

These are just some of the myths that exist regarding vaccines. There are many more that are more disease specific. Sometimes, people can just be plain wrong about the information. Other times, the myth has been so engrained in the culture and people. There is one very common myth that is going to be debunked in the next chapter. There is so much information that even the whole chapter doesn't encompass the entirety of this myth. Keep reading to find out which myth! You may have heard about it before.

Chapter 8: Autism

Autism. You've heard of it. It's actually called "Autism Spectrum Disorder" according to the DSM-V. What is it? It's a disorder in which the person typically has deficits in social cues, effective communication, and social interactions. This explanation, by the way, is very general and doesn't give many details. The disorder itself, as the official name encompasses, is a spectrum. The severity of the disorder varies greatly between individuals. The disorder is also very interesting as the symptoms also vary per person[4].

What causes autism? Do vaccines cause autism? The simple answer to the second question is "no." As for the first question, Autism Spectrum Disorder is one of those diseases that is not fully understood and needs more research. So, why are there so many people who believe that it does?

The root of this myth stems from an article that was published in *The Lancet*. The article was published by Dr. Andrew Wakefield in 1998. Dr. Wakefield was a well-known doctor in the United Kingdom. He worked at the Royal Free Hospital in London[1]. He had a pretty prestigious reputation. In fact, Dr. Wakefield was the doctor that was able to identify the cause of Crohn's disease[1]. He was very well known and his opinion was highly regard. Why wouldn't it be? He discovered the cause of a disease! Any scientist capable of that receives recognition and support. The support is usually so that they can further their research and try to get more significant findings. However, there may be some caveats to that belief.

The myth begins with his research. In one of his studies, Wakefield looked at twelve children with gastrointestinal problems as we all some neurological deficits. Of those children, eight of them had received the MMR vaccine. He noticed that within the intestines of these children, there was a high prevalence of the measles virus. From, that he concluded and published the article. The first and last pages of the article can be seen in figure 1 and figure 2. Take a very close look at the highlighted portion of figure 2. In his own article, he states "We did not prove an association between measles, mumps, and rubella vaccine and the syndrome described"[3]. He also continues to say "Published evidence is inadequate to show whether there is a change in incidence or a link with measles, mumps, and rubella vaccine"[3].

EARLY REPORT

Early report

Ileal-lymphoid-nodular hyperplasia, non-specific colitis, and pervasive developmental disorder in children

A J Wakefield, S H Murch, A Anthony, J Linnell, D M Casson, M Malik, M Berelowitz, A P Dhillon, M A Thomson, P Harvey, A Valentine, S E Davies, J A Walker-Smith

Summary

Background We investigated a consecutive series of children with chronic enterocolitis and regressive developmental disorder.

Methods 12 children (mean age 6 years [range 3–10], 11 boys) were referred to a paediatric gastroenterology unit with a history of normal development followed by loss of acquired skills, including language, together with diarrhoea and abdominal pain. Children underwent gastroenterological, neurological, and developmental assessment and review of developmental records. Ileocolonoscopy and biopsy sampling, magnetic-resonance imaging (MRI), electroencephalography (EEG), and lumbar puncture were done under sedation. Barium follow-through radiography was done where possible. Biochemical, haematological, and immunological profiles were examined.

Findings Onset of behavioural symptoms was associated, by the parents, with measles, mumps, and rubella vaccination in eight of the 12 children, with measles infection in one child, and otitis media in another. All 12 children had intestinal abnormalities, ranging from lymphoid nodular hyperplasia to aphthoid ulceration. Histology showed patchy chronic inflammation in the colon in 11 children and reactive ileal lymphoid hyperplasia in seven, but no granulomas. Behavioural disorders included autism (nine), disintegrative psychosis (one), and possible postviral or vaccinal encephalitis (two). There were no focal neurological abnormalities and MRI and EEG tests were normal. Abnormal laboratory results were significantly raised urinary methylmalonic acid compared with age-matched controls (p=0.003), low haemoglobin in four children, and low serum IgA in four children.

Interpretation We identified associated gastrointestinal disease and developmental regression in a group of previously normal children, which was generally associated in time with possible environmental triggers.

Lancet 1998; **351**: 637–41
See Commentary page

Inflammatory Bowel Disease Study Group, University Departments of Medicine and Histopathology (A J Wakefield FRCS, A Anthony MB, J Linnell PhD, A P Dhillon MRCPath, S E Davies MRCPath) and the University Departments of Paediatric Gastroenterology (S H Murch MB, D M Casson MRCP, M Malik MRCP, M A Thomson FRCP, J A Walker-Smith FRCP), Child and Adolescent Psychiatry (M Berelowitz FRCPsych), Neurology (P Harvey FRCP), and Radiology (A Valentine FRCR), Royal Free Hospital and School of Medicine, London NW3 2QG, UK

Correspondence to: Dr A J Wakefield

Introduction

We saw several children who, after a period of apparent normality, lost acquired skills, including communication. They all had gastrointestinal symptoms, including abdominal pain, diarrhoea, and bloating and, in some cases, food intolerance. We describe the clinical findings, and gastrointestinal features of these children.

Patients and methods

12 children, consecutively referred to the department of paediatric gastroenterology with a history of a pervasive developmental disorder with loss of acquired skills and intestinal symptoms (diarrhoea, abdominal pain, bloating and food intolerance), were investigated. All children were admitted to the ward for 1 week, accompanied by their parents.

Clinical investigations

We took histories, including details of immunisations and exposure to infectious diseases, and assessed the children. In 11 cases the history was obtained by the senior clinician (JW-S). Neurological and psychiatric assessments were done by consultant staff (PH, MB) with HMS-4 criteria.[1] Developmental histories included a review of prospective developmental records from parents, health visitors, and general practitioners. Four children did not undergo psychiatric assessment at admission; all had been assessed professionally elsewhere, so these assessments were used as the basis for their behavioural diagnosis.

After bowel preparation, ileocolonoscopy was performed by SHM or MAT under sedation with midazolam and pethidine. Paired frozen and formalin-fixed mucosal biopsy samples were taken from the terminal ileum; ascending, transverse, descending, and sigmoid colons, and from the rectum. The procedure was recorded by video or still images, and were compared with images of the previous seven consecutive paediatric colonoscopies (four normal colonoscopies and three on children with ulcerative colitis), in which the physician reported normal appearances in the terminal ileum. Barium follow-through radiography was possible in some cases.

Also under sedation, cerebral magnetic-resonance imaging (MRI), electroencephalography (EEG) including visual, brain stem auditory, and sensory evoked potentials (where compliance made these possible), and lumbar puncture were done.

Laboratory investigations

Thyroid function, serum long-chain fatty acids, and cerebrospinal-fluid lactate were measured to exclude known causes of childhood neurodegenerative disease. Urinary methylmalonic acid was measured in random urine samples from eight of the 12 children and 14 age-matched and sex-matched normal controls, by a modification of a technique described previously.[2] Chromatograms were scanned digitally on computer, to analyse the methylmalonic-acid zones from cases and controls. Urinary methylmalonic-acid concentrations in patients and controls were compared by a two-sample *t* test. Urinary creatinine was estimated by routine spectrophotometric assay.

Children were screened for antiendomyseal antibodies and boys were screened for fragile-X if this had not been done

THE LANCET • Vol 351 • February 28, 1998

Figure 1. First page of Wakefield's retracted article from *The Lancet* [3]

factors for Crohn's disease and persistent measles vaccine-strain virus infection has been found in children with autoimmune hepatitis.²¹

We did not prove an association between measles, mumps, and rubella vaccine and the syndrome described. Virological studies are underway that may help to resolve this issue.

If there is a causal link between measles, mumps, and rubella vaccine and this syndrome, a rising incidence might be anticipated after the introduction of this vaccine in the UK in 1988. Published evidence is inadequate to show whether there is a change in incidence²² or a link with measles, mumps, and rubella vaccine.²³ A genetic predisposition to autistic-spectrum disorders is suggested by over-representation in boys and a greater concordance rate in monozygotic than in dizygotic twins.¹⁵ In the context of susceptibility to infection, a genetic association with autism, linked to a null allele of the *complement (C) 4B* gene located in the class III region of the major-histocompatibility complex, has been recorded by Warren and colleagues.²⁴ *C4B*-gene products are crucial for the activation of the complement pathway and protection against infection: individuals inheriting one or two *C4B* null alleles may not handle certain viruses appropriately, possibly including attenuated strains.

Urinary methylmalonic-acid concentrations were raised in most of the children, a finding indicative of a functional vitamin B12 deficiency. Although vitamin B12 concentrations were normal, serum B12 is not a good measure of functional B12 status.²⁵ Urinary methylmalonic-acid excretion is increased in disorders such as Crohn's disease, in which cobalamin excreted in bile is not reabsorbed. A similar problem may have occurred in the children in our study. Vitamin B12 is essential for myelinogenesis in the developing central nervous system, a process that is not complete until around the age of 10 years. B12 deficiency may, therefore, be a contributory factor in the developmental regression.²⁶

We have identified a chronic enterocolitis in children that may be related to neuropsychiatric dysfunction. In most cases, onset of symptoms was after measles, mumps, and rubella immunisation. Further investigations are needed to examine this syndrome and its possible relation to this vaccine.

Addendum
Up to Jan 28, a further 40 patients have been assessed; 39 with the syndrome.

Contributors
A J Wakefield was the senior scientific investigator. S H Murch and M A Thomson did the colonoscopies. A Anthony, A P Dhillon, and S E Davies carried out the histopathology. J Linnell did the B12 studies. D M Casson and M Malik did the clinical assessment. M Berelowitz did the psychiatric assessment. P Harvey did the neurological assessment. A Valentine did the radiological assessment. JW-S was the senior clinical investigator.

Acknowledgments
This study was supported by the Special Trustees of Royal Free Hampstead NHS Trust and the Children's Medical Charity. We thank Francis Moll and the nursing staff of Malcolm Ward for their patience and expertise; the parents for providing the impetus for these studies; and Paula Domizio, Royal London NHS Trust, for providing control tissue samples.

References

1 Diagnostic and Statistical Manual of Mental Disorders (DSM-IV). 4th edn. Washington DC, USA: American Psychiatric Association, 1994.
2 Bhatt HR, Green A, Linnell JC. A sensitive micromethod for the routine estimations of methylmalonic acid in body fluids and tissues using thin-layer chromatography. *Clin Chem Acta* 1982; **118:** 311–21.
3 Fujimura Y, Kamoni R, Iida M. Pathogenesis of aphthoid ulcers in Crohn's disease: correlative findings by magnifying colonoscopy, electromicroscopy, and immunohistochemistry. *Gut* 1996; **38:** 724–32.
4 Asperger H. Die Psychopathologie des coeliakakranken kindes. *Ann Paediatr* 1961; **197:** 146–51.
5 Walker-Smith JA, Andrews J. Alpha-1 antitrypsin, autism and coeliac disease. *Lancet* 1972; **ii:** 883–84.
6 D'Eufemia P, Celli M, Finocchiaro R, et al. Abnormal intestinal permeability in children with autism. *Acta Paediatrica* 1996; **85:** 1076–79.
7 Panksepp J. A neurochemical theory of autism. *Trends Neurosci* 1979; **2:** 174–77.
8 Reichelt KL, Hole K, Hamberger A, et al. Biologically active peptide-containing fractions in schizophrenia and childhood autism. *Adv Biochem Psychopharmacol* 1981; **28:** 627.
9 Shattock P, Kennedy A, Rowell F, Berney TP. Role of neuropeptides in autism and their relation with classical neurotransmitters. *Brain Dysfunction* 1991; **3:** 328.
10 Waring RH, Ngong JM. Sulphate metabolism in allergy induced autism: relevance to disease aetiology. Conference proceedings, biological perspectives in autism, University of Durham, NAS 35–44.
11 Murch SH, MacDonald TT, Walker-Smith JA, Levin M, Lionetti P, Klein NJ. Disruption of sulphated glycosaminoglycans in intestinal inflammation. *Lancet* 1993; **341:** 711–41.
12 Warren RP, Singh VK. Elevated serotonin levels in autism: association with the major histocompatibility complex. *Neuropsychobiology* 1996; **34:** 72–75.
13 Lucarelli S, Frediani T, Zingoni AM, et al. Food allergy and infantile autism. *Panminerva Med* 1995; **37:** 137–41.
14 Rutter M, Taylor E, Hersov L. In: Child and adolescent psychiatry. 3rd edn. London: Blackwells Scientific Publications: 581–82.
15 Wing L. The Autistic Spectrum. London: Constable, 1996: 68–71.
16 Fudenberg HH. Dialysable lymphocyte extract (DLyE) in infantile onset autism: a pilot study. *Biotherapy* 1996; **9:** 13–17.
17 Gupta S. Immunology and immunologic treatment of autism. *Proc Natl Autism Assn Chicago* 1996; 455–60.
18 Miyamoto H, Tanaka T, Kitamoto N, Fukada Y, Takashi S. Detection of immunoreactive antigen with monoclonal antibody to measles virus in tissue from patients with Crohn's disease. *J Gastroenterol* 1995; **30:** 28–33.
19 Ekbom A, Wakefield AJ, Zack M, Adami H-O. Crohn's disease following early measles exposure. *Lancet* 1994; **344:** 508–10.
20 Thompson N, Montgomery S, Pounder RE, Wakefield AJ. Is measles vaccination a risk factor for inflammatory bowel diseases? *Lancet* 1995; **345:** 1071–74.
21 Kawashima H, Mori T, Takekuma K, Hoshika A, Hata A, Nakayama T. Polymerase chain reaction detection of the haemagglutinin gene from an attenuated measles strain in the peripheral mononuclear cells of children with autoimmune hepatitis. *Arch Virol* 1996; **141:** 877–84.
22 Wing L. Autism spectrum disorders: no evidence for or against an increase in prevalence. *BMJ* 1996; **312:** 327–28.
23 Miller D, Wadsworth J, Diamond J, Ross E. Measles vaccination and neurological events. *Lancet* 1997; **349:** 730–31.
24 Warren RP, Singh VK, Cole P, et al. Increased frequency of the null allele at the complement C4B locus in autism. *Clin Exp Immunol* 1991; **83:** 438–40.
25 England JM, Linnell JC. Problems with the serum vitamin B12 assay. *Lancet* 1980; **ii:** 1072–74.
26 Dillon MJ, England JM, Gompertz D, et al. Mental retardation, megaloblastic anaemic, homocysteine metabolism due to an error in B12 metabolism. *Clin Sci Mol Med* 1974; **47:** 43–61.

Figure 2. Last page of Wakefield's retracted article from *The Lancet* [3]

Wakefield made the point that there is no link between autism and the MMR vaccine. However, in press conferences after the article was published, Wakefield made claims that it did[2]. His claims and statements scared the public and the media ate everything up. Parents were terrified and didn't trust their doctors as much. Vaccine rates in the United Kingdom dropped significantly[1]. If Wakefield's study didn't show any link, why did he publicly condemn the MMR vaccine? Upon further speculation, there are many reasons why Wakefield was motivated to go against this vaccine. Also, remember, his study was incredibly flawed as well. At the time, it didn't matter much, everyone ate it up. With that, scientists raced off to find answers.

Let's look at his study first. Wakefield had only 12 children in his study. Each of these children, according to him, exhibited some form of autistic spectrum disorder. As mentioned, this study is much too small. There were also a few variables studied. Combined, with the small number of participants, there was a very high chance that some result was going to be statistically significant.

Wakefield was funded by a personal injury lawyer. His name was Richard Barr. This man was representing parents of autistic children who were suing pharmaceutical companies for compensation. He needed evidence to show that autism was caused by vaccines. In his world, it didn't matter if there was an actual link. All he needs to do is win his case in court. Six years after the article was published, an investigative reporter for the *Sunday Times* in London began exposing Wakefield. The reporter's name was Brian Deer and he sat down with Richard Horton, the editor-in-chief, and went over all the flaws and issues with Wakefield's study[1]. It turned out, that Wakefield supposedly received $100,000 for his study. At the time, that contribution was the highest funding he received for the study.

Later, during a court hearing, Wakefield was asked if he had received funding from Barr. He did not and could not deny that fact, however, he did try to say that he received around $50,000[1]. During investigation, it turned out Wakefield had actually received $800,000 for his study. He didn't even report who this money came from. Thus far, you can see that this man had failed to report where his money came from. He was not even honest about how much money he had received. That's not even the best part. He also failed to tell his collaborators. Upon hearing this, one of his collaborators found out and was furious. He and another nine co-authors of the paper retracted their names[1]. They had no idea he had received this money and they wanted no part in any of this story.

Now, this was not the only financial gain that Wakefield was getting from this myth. Prior to publishing his study, Wakefield had filed for patent application for a safer measles vaccine[1]. More specifically, his own measles vaccine. Yep. That's right. He was creating his own version of the vaccine and it was only for measles. There's obviously a problem here. There is already the MMR vaccine. This vaccine protects against three diseases and is already being used widely. If the MMR vaccine is still available, Wakefield's new vaccine has very little chance of being successful in the market. What can he do? The answer is simple, get rid of the MMR vaccine. That's basically what he tried to do. Wakefield's crusade against the MMR vaccine would be financially beneficial for him because his vaccine would be on the market. He had every reason to bad-mouth the MMR vaccine. If people stopped trusting it, it would go out of business and they would have to buy his vaccine.

For that reason, Wakefield was very much a proponent of vaccine safety. There's not a single doubt that many people would agree that vaccines need to be safe. However, he was proposing that the MMR vaccine was not safe at all. He claimed and explained to many people that the vaccines should be separated. Conveniently, he was also creating his own, safe version of the measles vaccine that people should trust. How is anyone supposed to trust that medical opinion if the speaker has ulterior motives?

The story doesn't stop there. Wakefield is also a very questionable man. His research was conducted without any approval. For any study, there has to be approval. The Ethical Practices Committee in England didn't approve his case. He failed to receive that approval but conducted his study any way. The approval is necessary to prevent people from being harmed for no reason. Without approval, Wakefield put 12 children under procedures that can cause major distress. These procedures included biopsies and spinal as the green high-lighted region indicates in figure 1 above[3]. He literally did not have permission to put these children through those procedures. They can be harmful. They put the patient at many risks. How can someone do any of those procedures knowing they do not have the approval? This instance isn't the only questionable part about Wakefield's scientific practices.

Another important point about his study is that five of his participants were clients of Richard Barr[1]. That's right. His study purposefully had clients of the personal injury lawyer that was paying him. Essentially, this study had handpicked participants that skewed the data. For a scientific study to be considered reliable and true, participants must be chosen at random. The term "random" is actually very confusing for many students when they first learn it. When choosing at random, a researcher isn't supposed to find a random place and pick a random group of people. That isn't what makes it random. A study must have a group of participants that represent the population well. Picking participants at random means that the study was not tampered with and that there were no biases. The main point of scientific studies is to see what happens and try to limit as many influencers as possible. Hand-picking five of the participants instantly shows that the study is unreliable in the scientific community.

Not only did Wakefield have a bias in creating his research. It was also found that many of the children who were claimed to have deficits, actually did not have any. The parents of these children stepped up years later. They said their children did not actually have some of symptoms that Wakefield had originally claimed[2]. Aside from making false claims. Wakefield was also aware that his results did not show what they claimed they did? What do I mean?

During Dan Burton's congressional committee hearing, more controversial [handwritten: refused to put his name on anything] information regarding Wakefield's was brought out of the shadows. Wakefield's research assistant, Nicholas Chadwick had testified against him. Who's this Chadwick guy? Chadwick was the research assistant who personally tested the biopsies of each child from the MMR study. He personally did the PCR test for the measles RNA from each sample. He even said that all his results were negative. He mentioned getting false positives but had reported all the findings as negative to Wakefield. Wakefield on the other hand completely ignored him. In fact, he was fully aware his data did not show any evidence to support his hypothesis. Despite the glaring evidence, he went ahead and lied about the data. From these events, Chadwick refused to put his name on anything with the PCR data as it was poor practice[1].

As you can see, Andrew Wakefield literally fabricated his data. That, by the way, is a huge no-no in the scientific community. It is fraud. For the future researchers reading this book, here is some advice: NEVER LIE OR MAKE UP YOUR OWN DATA. NEVER. DON'T DO IT. Seriously though, stay honest, you could hurt more people around you than just yourself if you lie.

To continue discussing Wakefield and his questionable characteristics. At a child's birthday party, Wakefield decided to draw blood from the children and paid them for it[1]. There are very clearly many reasons why this is wrong. First of all, there is no approval whatsoever for him to conduct this research. Second, he probably didn't obtain permission from these children's parents. Third, who in the right mind would ever draw blood at a birthday party? If this man is capable of so many unethical behaviors, why are we trusting his medical advice?

The General Medical Council in London took away Andrew Wakefield's medical license in September 2005. They stated that he had several counts of misconduct and I've already explained each of these misconducts already. As a result, this man is no longer allowed to practice medicine. Therefore, his medical advice probably shouldn't be taken any more. Right? After the United Kingdom stripped him of his license, Wakefield moved to Texas[1].

Some of his most recent activity involves meeting with President Trump. This meeting caused an uproar and some major concern on social media[5]. Why? Someone who lost their medical license probably shouldn't be dispensing advice regarding public health policy, right? However, it's unlikely that Trump will change major public health policy as politicians and scientists would argue against him[6]. His beliefs do give anti-vaccine activists the energy and support to strongly ignore the science and continue claiming that MMR causes autism[6]. Essentially, having a major political leader with these beliefs can strengthen a cultural belief even if he doesn't change any actual policy. He is a symbol who just perpetuates misinformation.

Let's recap. Dr. Wakefield was a well-known physician that was held in high regard. He published a small and unreliable study. In his own publication, pointed out that there was no link between the vaccine and the disorder. Despite his own publication, he publicly claimed that the MMR vaccine caused autism at a press conference. From this claim, so many people became concerned. The media took the information and ran with it to create their insanely biased opinions. Many scientists looked into whether the vaccine did cause autism. Many parents stopped vaccinating their children with the MMR vaccine until it was proven to be safe. Many parents with children with autism latched onto this information as they were desperately looking for answers.

For his own gain, Wakefield was perpetuating the idea that autism was caused by the MMR vaccine because he was paid by a personal injury lawyer and he was trying to sell his own measles vaccine. His medical license was in question and the United Kingdom took it away. This man has conducted many unethical and questionable actions. Yet, he is still highly revered by many people. He still has many followers and people who believe in him. In fact, there are many conspiracy theorists who are convinced that the government is trying to hide information.

As Andrew Wakefield and his infamous autism and vaccine debacle started to die down, another vaccine myth was created. As the MMR vaccine myth slowly died down, mercury gained the spotlight. Sometime in the 1997, there was a congressman that was devoted to improving the environment[1]. He was very concerned about the presence of mercury in the environment. From his concern, the FDA went on a mission to determine how much mercury is actually in certain products[1]. This very well-intentioned concern begins the story of how thimerosal and mercury poisoning get involved with the vaccine and autism myth.

But first, where does mercury come into play with autism? There was a vaccine ingredient known as thimerosal. It was a preservative that was used in inactivated vaccines so that unwanted bacteria would not grow inside the vaccines. Thimerosal was created by a pharmaceutical company that was known as Eli Lilly[1]. This company took ethylmercury and combined it with thiosalicylate to create thimerosal[1]. That's where the mercury comes in. Ethylmercury. This compound was confused with methylmercury.

What's the difference? The difference is that ethylmercury has one more carbon than the methylmercury[2]. However, that distinction is very important. Methylmercury is found in the environment. It's pretty dangerous. It causes the major defects. This compound takes longer to excrete from the body and therefore can cause more damage. In contrast, ethylmercury is a little bit of a larger compound. Since it is larger, it is excreted out of the body more quickly and is less likely to cause damage[1].

Don't believe me that two similarly sounding compounds can be different. Let's think about another example. Alright, you're at this awesome party. It's dark. There's loud music. There are flashing lights everywhere. Someone comes up and offers you two drinks. One drink contains methanol and one drink contains ethanol. Which one do you choose?

I sure hope you paid close attention to your Alcohol Ed module before you came to college and chose the ethanol (I'll personally be very sad if you chose the methanol). Just as ethanol is safe for you to drink while methanol would cause blindness, ethylmercury is safer than methylmercury.

What happened with thimerosal then? The FDA looked at how much mercury was in certain products. They found that there was ethylmercury in vaccines. The FDA only had research and data on methylmercury[1]. There were no guidelines regarding ethylmercury. Despite this lack of data, the FDA held a meeting to discuss the mercury issues. At this meeting was Dr. Neal Halsey[1]. From this meeting, Dr. Neal Halsey became very passionate about removing mercury from vaccines. He had very good intentions. He didn't want children to get sick. He truly meant well. Except, the entire meeting he had gone to had applied the data from methylmercury to ethylmercury which does not provide an accurate picture.

That distinction didn't really matter because after the meeting, Dr. Halsey was on a precautionary policy crusade. He was determined to remove thimerosal from vaccines just as a precaution to keep children safe. He was very adamant and hasty. In fact, many members of the CDC, AAP, and National Vaccine Advisory Committee did not agree with him[1]. They didn't really want to remove thimerosal as there was no clear indication that it caused any harm. Dr. Halsey was still very zealous. He put together teleconferences and pushed for change and decisions.

Ultimately, he got what he wanted but at a price. The policy was created. The entire precaution was confusing and unnecessary. It didn't make much sense. The chemical was removed because of the mercury. Except, scientists didn't know if the mercury in vaccines was harmful. As a result, the public was confused because why would the government take it out if it's not harmful? They would only want to take it out because it must be harmful? Maybe the government is just lying?

The removal of the thimerosal as a precautionary step was, as mentioned, not favored by everyone. There were members of the CDC who actually predicted that the removal will cause parents to blame thimerosal for autism. In fact, this quote can be found in *Autism's False Prophets*:

> "It is possible that many children born in the 1990s who have serious disorders of unknown etiology will now blame mercury in vaccines for their illnesses. This is particularly likely for illnesses that appear to be increasing, such as autism".[1]

This quote describes exactly what had happened. As MMR associations to autism slowly waned away, thimerosal received the blame. However, the truth would prevail. The removal of thimerosal created a natural experiment. Basically, no vaccines contained this compound which meant that babies born after this policy would never have any in their bodies. If thimerosal caused autism, there would be a decrease in cases of autism. If thimerosal didn't cause autism, the amount of cases would remain the same. This natural experiment would take about six years as autism is typically diagnosed around that age. The six years passed and cases of autism actually increased. At first, there was a decrease but more years passed and it became clear that thimerosal did not cause autism[1].

There is another piece of evidence that shows very clearly that thimerosal could not cause autism. The symptoms of mercury poisoning are the complete opposite of autism[2]. Two scientists decided to compare and contrast children with mercury poisoning and children with autism. They found that children with autism had on average larger heads while children with mercury poisoning had smaller heads. They also found that children with mercury poisoning had vision problems while children with autism did not. Children with autism were usually "socially aloof" whereas children with mercury poisoning were found to be psychotic[1]. These disorders are very clearly polar opposites from each other.

Despite the evidence, there are many people who offer "cures" to autism. There are so many people but I'm only going to focus on Jenny McCarthy and the Geiers. Jenny McCarthy, formerly a *Playboy* model, is a very vocal anti-vaccine advocate. She dropped out of nursing school to become a model so she doesn't really have medical expertise[7]. Her story is that her son was perfectly fine but after receiving a vaccine, she believed he got autism from receiving the shot[7]. McCarthy claims that the life in her son's eyes disappeared and she had lost him. This description, by the way, can be seen as very hurtful to many people in the autism community and their families[7]. After all, the disorder is a disability that many people live with.

Jenny McCarthy claims she cured her son's autism through diet, supplements and other strange products[7]. She even wrote a book describing the cures. Her main message is that mothers know best and doctors are untrustworthy. In her defense, she probably did have a condescending doctor who hurt her feelings. She is one of many people who claim to have found a cure. The only problem is that there isn't a cure. As I mentioned, she also doesn't have medical expertise so I think most of her products probably just empty out wallets.

Moving onto other anti-vaccine activists, we have the Geiers. The Geiers are a father and son duo[1]. They both have backgrounds in science, but their fields of study are not specialized in immunology, epidemiology, microbiology or any other vaccine related field. Initially, they didn't believe that thimerosal was causing autism, However, they decided to look into the VAERS for their data. What is VAERS? It stands for Vaccine Adverse Event Reporting System[2]. This database relies on people self-reporting their adverse effects. There isn't a medical professional inputting this data and there is no screening. It is basically an unfiltered method for people to report whatever they think is an adverse effect to the vaccine[2]. The system initially had the right intentions. After a while, the CDC realized there needed to be some sort of regulation yet, it's not regularly checked. For that reason, someone could report that the vaccine caused them to become a mermaid and it would be real evidence until taken down.

Back to the Geiers, the two are known for creating treatments to cure autism. One treatment is chelation. This therapy takes dangerous chemicals and injects them straight into the body[1]. The mercury in the body binds to these chemicals and leaves. This therapy is very dangerous as deaths can occur. In fact, in there was a boy who died of chelation therapy. This boy's mother was trying her best to take care of him. The boy's name was Tariq Nadama. He was five years old. His mother took him to a DAN doctor. DAN stands for "Defeat Autism Now"[1]. These doctors basically perform treatments that supposedly cure autism. In Tariq's case, a doctor injected EDTA into his blood. The doctor needed another doctor's assistance in getting the boy to stop fussing. Then, his mother noticed something was wrong. Tariq's blood pressure dropped. An ambulance was called, Tariq arrived at the hospital. The doctors initially announced that he had died of a heart attack. A pathologist later determined that the EDTA caused Tariq to die from very low levels of calcium. It turns out that EDTA binds to calcium, not mercury. The doctor who did all of this was charged with involuntary manslaughter and reckless endangerment. Although his charges were dropped, doctors shouldn't be getting criminal charges in the first place[1].

The Geiers also created their own drug known as Lupron. This drug stops testosterone production. In my opinion, a red flag should go up right there. A drug that stops testosterone production? Children, especially young boys, need testosterone. Although Lupron disrupts important metabolic pathways, it was still patented and sold. The sad part is that during this time, there was minimal research and it could potentially cause sterility in these young boys. Among these treatments, are many others. There are many industries that sells supplements, diets, and other products that "cure" autism. Each of these fake cures provide false hope to parents. Some of these parents are very desperate and look for any shred of hope. They have good intentions and want the best for their children. For instance, Tariq mother definitely didn't want her son to die. She just wanted his life to be easier. As you can see, the treatments that are out there are incredibly dangerous and many parents are being misled.

Wakefield and the Geiers are not the only scientists who supported the claim that the MMR vaccine caused autism. Some other scientists included the following: Vijendra Singh, Walter Spitzer, Hisash Kawashima, Kenneth Aitken, and many more[1]. However, there were also many scientists who showed that the vaccines do not cause autism. A team from Helsinki University in Finland studied the records of 2 million children and saw no link between autism and the MMR vaccine. From Boston University School of Medicine, researchers looked at medical records of 3 million children and noticed that autism rates were increasing but not due to vaccines. From the Department of Health Services in Berkley California, Loring Dales and Natalie Smith found that autism was increasing and had nothing to do with the MMR vaccine. There are so many more studies and so much more research showing that MMR did not cause autism[1].

Despite all the research, the myths persist and more have been formed. For instance, there is a myth that thimerosal was used in MMR vaccines and those vaccines cause autism. However, the MMR vaccine is a live-attenuated vaccine which means it never needed thimerosal. It never contained thimerosal yet, there were and are people convinced that it did. It's probably because these two myths combined to create a new one. The creation of this myth shows how easy misinformation can occur and perpetuate.

As you can see, there is so much behind the vaccine and autism myths and so many health care professionals, researchers, politicians, celebrities and members of the media are involved. There is also ample evidence against the vaccine and autism myths. Who do you think should we believe?

Chapter 9: Ingredients

"All things are poison, and nothing is without poison; only the dose permits something not to be poisonous" –Paracelsus[1]

Okay, so we've already talked about vaccines and the science behind them. Now let's discuss what's in them. We know that the vaccine has to contain the antigens that were mentioned earlier. That is absolutely true. Scientists also have to formulate these shots so that they are effective and do not go bad. Yes, vaccines can go bad. Some need some bits of preservatives and careful storage. Actually, no, some need many preservatives and for a good reason. No one wants to have a spoiled vaccine injected straight into their blood. Since there are many ingredients in all the vaccines that exist, the ingredients can be placed into four categories of ingredients. These ingredients are divided into adjuvants, antigens, fluids and preservatives/stabilizers[1].

[vaccine ingredients]

Adjuvants

These are compounds that enhance the vaccine's ability to create an immune response. The adjuvants in vaccines help the body create a stronger response to the antigens[1]. These compounds also make it easier for vaccine manufacturers to use less of the pathogen. In other words, these chemicals elicit a better response with fewer antigens.

Antigens

As mentioned earlier, antigens are the proteins that the body can recognize as foreign. The antigens that are used in vaccines are weakened viruses, killed viruses, specific pieces of viruses, and pieces of bacterial components or secretions[1]. The antigens are what create the immune response and are the key ingredient to the vaccines.

Fluids

The fluids are pretty self-explanatory. The vaccine manufacturers need a way to get the antigens inside the body. The fluids that are used for vaccines just serve as a mode of transport for the antigens[1]. The most common fluid used in most vaccines is sterilized water (not just normal tap water but sterilized water)[1]. *[most common]*

Preservatives/Stabilizers

The preservatives basically stop the vaccine solutions from going bad. It is very possible for bacterial growth to occur in vaccines. For that reason, chemicals are added to keep vaccines from becoming harmful. It makes sense, you wouldn't want to inject another pathogen into the body while trying to gain protection from another one. Preservatives and stabilizers are also important for prolonging the shelf-life. Without preservatives, manufacturers would have to make more vaccines and these vaccines could end up costing a lot more money[1].

On the following page, there is a table that lists common vaccine ingredients in their specific categories. Some ingredients are used for manufacturing while other ingredients are in the vaccines. For instance, albumin and yeast protein are sometimes left over in trace amounts in vaccines as they are typically grown in cell cultures. Some cells that are usually used in the culturing process are eggs cells and human fetal embryo fibroblast cells (these are from fetal tissue from two elected abortions from the 1960s)[2].

Table 1. Common Vaccine Ingredients Categorized [1]

Antigens	Fluids	Preservatives/Stabilizers	Adjuvants
Killed Viruses	Distilled/Sterilized Water	Formaldehyde/ Formalin	Aluminum Hydroxide,
Partial Bacteria		Monosodium Glutamate (MSG) Neomycin	Aluminum hydroxyphosphate sulfate
Partial Viruses		Phenoxyethanol, 2-Phenoyxethanol Polymyxin B Sorbitol	Monophoshoryl lipid A
Weak Live Viruses		Sucrose Gelatin Amino Acids Phosphate Buffers	Squalene
Bacterial Toxoids		Polysorbate 80 Sodium Chloride	

In the table above, there is a very large list of preservatives and stabilizers. What are some of those chemicals? Formaldehyde/formalin is an organic compound that is actually naturally found in the human body[1]. This ingredient is highly controversial and I will discuss it in further detail a little later. Monosodium glutamate (MSG) is actually a flavor enhancing salt that is used in some foods (such as Chinese food)[1]. MSG can naturally be found in foods such as peas and grape juice. There is actually about 0.200mg per 100g and 0.258mg of MSG per 100g found in peas and grape juice respectively[1].

The next ingredient, neomycin, is an antibiotic so it prevents the growth of other bacteria in the vaccine vial. The phenoxyethanol/ 2-phenoxyethanol is a preservative. This compound can be found in sunscreen, perfume and some cosmetics. Polymyxin B is another antibiotic that is used to prevent growth of bacteria. There are also sorbitol and sucrose which are natural sweeteners. The sorbitol is a preservative while the sucrose helps the vaccine remain potent. Gelatin is used as a stabilizer and is found in foods such as Jell-O. Gelatin is a collagen-derivative which basically makes things gelatinous[1].

There are also amino acids. If you remind from your biology class, amino acids are the building blocks of proteins. They are incredibly important for human nutrition (think about all the body builders drinking those protein shakes). Amino acids, specifically glycine, are used a stabilizer in vaccines. Phosphate buffers are used as a stabilizer. The phosphate buffers are a family of compounds that help maintain the pH (the acidity/basicity) of the vaccine. Polysorbate 80 acts as an emulsifier and as a solubilizer. An emulsifier is a compound that keeps a liquid from separating. Essentially, this compound tries to prevent the vaccine from separating like when oil is dropped in water. Polysorbate 80 also acts as solubilizer in vaccines because it keeps the ingredients mixed together. Sodium chloride, also known as table salt, stabilizes that cellular environments of the vaccines. Those are the functions of many of the preservatives and stabilizers that are used in vaccines[1].

There are also some compounds used ad adjuvants. Common adjuvants include aluminum salts which are discussed later. There are also monophosphoryl lipid A and squalene[3]. Monophosphoryl lipid A is a modified form of a sugar compound found in bacterial cell walls[5]. This compound is detoxified and used as an adjuvant[5]. Squalene is an oil-in-water emulsion[3]. This compound is typically taken from fish oils. In the United States, vaccines use shark liver oil for this compound. Squalene is also a compound that human livers make naturally. It can be found in the bloodstream as part of cholesterol synthesis[3].

Over the years, there have been many ingredients have caused major concern for people. The following list goes through a few of the controversial ingredients:

Formaldehyde controversial

You may have heard of formaldehyde. If you haven't, it's used to preserve dead bodies. Why is it used in vaccines? When creating inactivated vaccines, such as the influenza vaccine, scientists use a form of formaldehyde to "kill" the virus. It effectively damages the virus enough so that it can no longer reproduce. The protein structures are still recognizable. The formaldehyde also inhibits the growth of harmful bacteria (similar to the antibiotics). The compound also preserves the efficacy of the vaccines.

Formaldehyde is also naturally produced in your body in small quantities. It is specifically produced when your cells replicate using DNA synthesis[7]. In fact, at a given time, there is 25ug of formaldehyde for 1mL of blood[7]. Now, I'm not saying that formaldehyde isn't bad for your body. High levels of formaldehyde can damage DNA and create cancerous mutations to cells that are in a lab setting. However, the tiny amounts found inside a vaccine is not going to damage your body significantly. Repeated exposure, for extended and prolonged amounts of time are more likely to have those effects on the body. Not only does your body produce this compound, it is also found in many everyday items you wouldn't think of. One of my favorite examples is one that involves bananas. You probably didn't know this but bananas contain formaldehyde. Imagine three medium sized bananas, how much formaldehyde do you think is in them? There are about 16.3 grams of formaldehyde in three medium-sized bananas[1]. Personally, when I make banana bread, I use three medium sized bananas. Vaccines, however, contain much less than that. For instance, most vaccines contain about 1.2mg of formaldehyde[1]. Which do you think is more likely to pose harm?

Aluminum

Aluminum is used in vaccines as an adjuvant. The aluminum is found in the form of salts and they basically make the vaccine more effective which is exactly what we want. However, some parents have panicked that the aluminum in vaccines was going to cause their children neurological deficits. Let's think about this for a moment. Yes, aluminum is a neurotoxin[4].
However, the amount in vaccines is much, much too small to even cause that sort of damage. Aluminum is also a very common element and can be found in many everyday food items. Adults consume 7 to 9mg of aluminum every day[4]. Aluminum can be found in fruits and vegetables, as well as cereals, nuts, dairy products and baby formula. In comparison to the 7-9mg, vaccines contain between 0.01mg to 0.90mg per dose of aluminum[4]. That is an insanely large difference.

A review study conducted by Jefferson et al, found that there was no evidence that aluminum salts can cause serious long-term effects or adverse reactions. This study looked at 23 reports of studies and determined if there were any consequences between the aluminum adjuvants and adverse effects[6]. The study concluded that there was no evidence to support that aluminum adjuvants are harmful[6].

Some people make the argument that there is a difference between injecting something directly into the blood versus orally consuming it through the mouth. In both cases, the substance will end up in the bloodstream no matter what, that's just how our bodies work. The tiny amount of aluminum used as adjuvants are very unlikely to cause damage to a person when it is injected into the bloodstream.

Hydrochloric Acid

Hydrochloric acid is used in the manufacturing of some vaccines. The acid is very strong. It is naturally found in your stomach acid. In terms of vaccines, the acid is used to stabilize the pH of the solutions. The hydrochloric acid dissociates so that it is not harmful to the body. Remember in your high school chemistry class when your teacher discussed acids and bases? HCl is a strong acid that breaks down completely in water so that it cannot harm you. If you can't remember your high school chemistry class, that's perfectly fine! The acid is only harmful if it is intact. In water, it breaks down. The HCl is put in some fluid, typically sterilized water, and therefore cannot harm anyone. Without the HCl, the vaccine, specifically DTaP, would be dangerous to inject into people[1].

[handwritten annotation: b/c it completely dissociates]

It is important to remember that some ingredients have scary names. However, many of the foods we eat everyday also contain compounds with weird and long names. For instance, read the ingredients for the following foods and beverages (try to guess the foods).

Food Item #1

INGREDIENTS: NONFAT MILK, LACTOSE, VEGETABLE OIL (PALM OLEIN, COCONUT, SOY, AND HIGH OLEIC SUNFLOWER OILS), WHEY PROTEIN CONCENTRATE, AND LESS THAN 2%: GALACTOOLIGOSACCHARIDES*, POLYDEXTROSE*, MORTIERELLA ALPINA OIL·, CRYPTHECODINIUM COHNII OIL·, CALCIUM CARBONATE, POTASSIUM CITRATE, FERROUS SULFATE, POTASSIUM CHLORIDE, MAGNESIUM OXIDE, SODIUM CHLORIDE, ZINC SULFATE, CUPRIC SULFATE, MANGANESE SULFATE, POTASSIUM IODIDE, SODIUM SELENITE, SOY LECITHIN, CHOLINE CHLORIDE, ASCORBIC ACID, NIACINAMIDE, CALCIUM PANTOTHENATE, VITAMIN A PALMITATE, VITAMIN B_{12}, VITAMIN D_3, RIBOFLAVIN, THIAMIN HYDROCHLORIDE, VITAMIN B_6 HYDROCHLORIDE, FOLIC ACID, VITAMIN K_1, BIOTIN, INOSITOL, VITAMIN E ACETATE, NUCLEOTIDES (CYTIDINE 5'-MONOPHOSPHATE, DISODIUM URIDINE 5'-MONOPHOSPHATE, ADENOSINE 5'-MONOPHOSPHATE, DISODIUM GUANOSINE 5'-MONOPHOSPHATE), TAURINE, L-CARNITINE.

*A TYPE OF PREBIOTIC
·A SOURCE OF ARACHIDONIC ACID (ARA)
·A SOURCE OF DOCOSAHEXAENOIC ACID (DHA)

Please refer to your product packaging for the most accurate information.

Last Updated: 5/18/17

Figure 1. List of Ingredients [2]

Food Item #2

Ingredients: Corn, Vegetable Oil (Sunflower, Canola, and/or Corn Oil), Maltodextrin (Made From Corn), Salt, Cheddar Cheese (Milk, Cheese Cultures, Salt, Enzymes), Whey, Monosodium Glutamate, Buttermilk, Romano Cheese (Part-Skim Cow's Milk, Cheese Cultures, Salt, Enzymes), Whey Protein Concentrate, Onion Powder, Corn Flour, Natural and Artificial Flavor, Dextrose, Tomato Powder, Lactose, Spices, Artificial Color (Including Yellow 6, Yellow 5, and Red 40), Lactic Acid, Citric Acid, Sugar, Garlic Powder, Skim Milk, Red and Green Bell Pepper Powder, Disodium Inosinate, and Disodium Guanylate.
CONTAINS MILK INGREDIENTS.

Figure 2. List of Ingredients[10]

Food Item #3

INGREDIENTS: AQUA (84%), **SUGARS (10%)** (FRUCTOSE (48%), GLUCOSE (40%), SUCROSE (2%)), FIBRE E460 (2.4%), **AMINO ACIDS (<1%)** (GLUTAMIC ACID (23%), ASPARTIC ACID (18%), LEUCINE (17%), ARGININE (8%), ALANINE (4%), VALINE (4%), GLYCINE (4%), PROLINE (4%), ISOLEUCINE (3%), SERINE (3%), THREONINE (3%), PHENYLALANINE (2%), LYSINE (2%), METHIONINE (2%), TYROSINE (1%), HISTIDINE (1%), CYSTINE (1%), TRYPTOPHAN (<1%)), **FATTY ACIDS (<1%)** (OMEGA-6 FATTY ACID: LINOLEIC ACID (30%), OMEGA-3 FATTY ACID: LINOLENIC ACID (19%), OLEIC ACID (18%), PALMITIC ACID (6%), STEARIC ACID (2%), PALMITOLEIC ACID (<1%)), ASH (<1%), PHYTOSTEROLS, OXALIC ACID, E300, E306 (TOCOPHEROL), THIAMIN, **COLOURS** (E163a, E163b, E163e, E163f, E160a) **FLAVOURS** (ETHYL ETHANOATE, 3-METHYL BUTYRALDEHYDE, 2-METHYL BUTYRALDEHYDE, PENTANAL, METHYLBUTYRATE, OCTENE, HEXANAL, DECANAL, 3-CARENE, LIMONENE, STYRENE, NONANE, ETHYL-3-METHYLBUTANOATE, NON-1-ENE, HEXAN-2-ONE, HYDROXYLINALOOL, LINALOOL, TERPINYL ACETATE, CARYOPHYLLENE, ALPHA-TERPINEOL, ALPHA-TERPINENE, 1,8-CINEOLE, CITRAL, BENZALDEHYDE), METHYLPARABEN, 1510, E300, E440, E421 and **FRESH AIR** (E941, E948, E290).

Figure 3. List of Ingredients [11]

What are your guesses for each food label? Drum rolls, please. The first food label is Enfamil which is a baby formula. The second food label display the ingredients of Doritos. Before moving on, let's take a look at the ingredients. In figure 1, one can see many chemical compound names. For instance, there are galactoolgosaccharides[2]. What even are those? There is manganese sulfate as well as calcium pantothenate? Those things are in baby formula? What about the Doritos? In figure 2, there are more food items such as corn and Romano cheese[10]. However, there's our lovely friend monosodium glutamate (one of the preservatives in vaccines). Now, what's the last food? It has insane words such as 3-methyl butyraldehyde and oxalic acid[11]. What food has those scary ingredients? The answer? Blueberries? Don't believe me? Look at the figure 4 below.

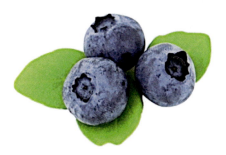

Figure 4. Blueberry Food Label[11]

The figure above, figure 4, is from a chemistry teacher's blog. His name is James Kennedy[11]. He creates food labels of foods that people normally eat to show how they all have scary chemical names. He also makes a point to label each ingredient list with "All-Natural" at the top[11]. His point is that these natural foods that people eat everyday are completely safe but the chemical names of compounds can be very misleading. What's the main point of all these examples? To point out that everyday food items that are made for babies, all-natural foods and some popular junk foods all have scary ingredients. However, they're consumed every day and people typically aren't harmed.

Another important note I would to make relates back to the quote that opens this chapter. This quote is from Paracelsus and it goes "All things are poison, and nothing is without poison; only the dose permits something not to be poisonous"[1]. By this point, most people have probably heard that if they drink too much water, they can drown their cells. However, there are many other foods and beverages that people consume that pose harm.

One of the most popular beverages that can cause some serious harm is alcohol. As a college student, many of you may decide to partake in social drinking. Many adults also decide to enjoy a glass of wine every once in a while. Just a reminder, ethanol is toxic to the human body. It is basically a poison and people actively choose to drink it. You may be thinking, "nah, there's no way." Nope, your liver works to detoxify your body of the alcohol. That being said, how much a person consumes and how quickly determines whether it will be poisonous or not. Having one drink an hour is certainly not dangerous for most people. Having six drinks in half an hour is a whole different story. There are horror stories out there about consuming too much alcohol. The bottom line is that too much of one thing can be dangerous. The dose is extremely important.

Now, let's extend that concept to vaccines. The dose for many of the ingredients in vaccines are in teeny, tiny quantities. In fact, most of these ingredients are present in microliters[1]. Through my personal lab experience, most of these quantities are smaller than a little drop of liquid. Let's put these amounts into perspective. The following image, figure 5 shows the relative comparisons of some common metric liquid units.

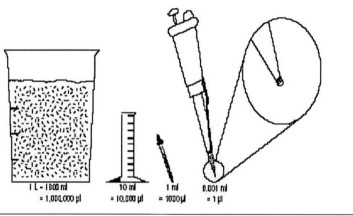

Figure 5. Liquid metric unit comparisons [8]

As you can see, the largest quantity in the figure is the liter. The smallest is a microliter. The microliter is basically a little drop. The quantities found in vaccines range between the milliliters and the microliters. If those quantities still don't make much sense, that's perfectly fine! Think about a penny. A penny is about 2.5g[1]. Vaccines have ingredients that are usually measured in milligrams (mg) or in micrograms (mcg). A milligram is about the weight of a grain of sand and the microgram is much smaller[1]. Essentially, the amounts of the ingredients in vaccines are very small, to the point that the human eye can have some difficulty locating it.

Overall, the main point of this chapter is that the dose is the key to understanding vaccine ingredients. Any of the ingredients can be considered poisonous given the wrong dose.

Chapter 10: Create the Herd

Herd immunity is a concept that relies on high vaccination rates within a population. The idea is that within a population of people, those who are capable of getting vaccinated can protect those who cannot get vaccinated. That explanation is slightly complicated but makes sense after a few attempts.

Let's take a look at a simplified example using measles. There are two populations. Each population has about the same number of people. Each population has people who are immunocompromised and for medical purposes are incapable of receiving vaccines. Population A enforces vaccination. Population B doesn't enforce vaccination. As a result, Population A has a higher vaccination rate than Population B. A family from a foreign country visits each of these populations. One member of the family is sick and brings measles along.

When the family enters Population A, many people are vaccinated. They interact with these people and are capable of preventing the disease from infecting their vulnerable population. The people who are vaccinated act as a barrier to the people who are unvaccinated or immunocompromised. Since most of the population is protected against the disease, the measles virus is less likely to spread.

When the family enters Population B, most people are unvaccinated and are infected with the disease. The disease spreads quickly amongst the population and infects everyone who was unvaccinated including those who are immunocompromised. As a result, there are many deaths and a large epidemic. Since these people were mostly unvaccinated, there were more people who contracted and spread the disease. The virus had enough people to spread between.

What happened? In Population A, enough people were vaccinated in order to prevent the spread of disease between most people. In Population B, there were not enough vaccinated people and the disease was able to spread. In figure 1, below, the image shows three populations. Population B is represented by the top group while population is represented by the bottom group. The middle group shows a group that has a mixture of vaccination rates.

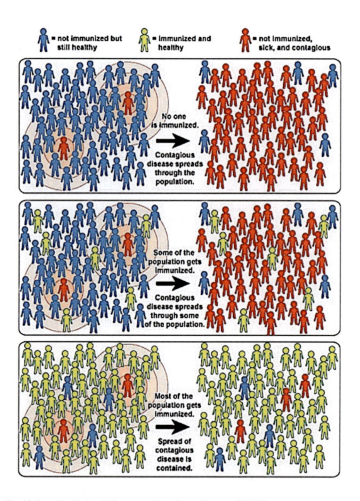

Photo credit: Courtesy: The National Institute of Allergy and Infectious Disease (NIAID)

Figure 1. Herd immunity[2]

To see herd immunity in action, you can actually look at *The Guardian's* animation with this link right here: https://www.theguardian.com/society/ng-interactive/2015/feb/05/-sp-watch-how-measles-outbreak-spreads-when-kids-get-vaccinated.

Herd immunity does not promise that everyone will remain safe. Sometimes a disease is still able to find its way through a population and harm an immunocompromised individual. However, the concept, when implemented properly, can protect many people.

As mentioned before, there are many people in the world who are unable to get vaccinated. These people are left vulnerable and susceptible to disease. They are considered immunocompromised. You may be that person or know someone close to you who is considered immunocompromised. Who exactly fits into this category? The geriatric population (old people), transplant patients, patients with autoimmune diseases, infants, cancer patients and pregnant women. immunocompromised

If herd immunity is important, how can a population achieve it? Herd immunity has many different factors that play a role. The first part of it to understand is that each disease has its own herd immunity threshold (HIT) for susceptible. This threshold depends on the disease's communicability, the type of pathogen (virus or bacterium), transmission and who it infects. Each of these factors is determined by R_0 (pronounced R "naught"). This symbol represents the basic reproduction number of the disease. The basic reproduction number shows how many cases of a disease one person could create in a fully susceptible population.

For example, the R_0 of measles, a highly contagious disease, is between 12 and 16. This number indicates that one person could spread the disease, on average, to 12 to 16 more people. (Keep in mind that the 12 to 16 is an average, depending on the source and algorithm, the number may be different). As you can probably tell, measles is one of those diseases that really requires a high herd immunity threshold[1].

In figure 2 below, the herd immunity diagram has an R_0 of four. In case A, there are only susceptible people in the population. In case B, there is a mixture of immune and susceptible people within the population. In case A, the first person easily transmits the disease to four people. Then those four people transmit the disease to another four people each (a total of 16). In the entire population, there are 21 people who now have the unknown disease.

In contrast, in case B, the infected person only manages to transmit the disease to one susceptible person because the other three are immune. That one person encounters four people and only one of them gets infected. In this population, 15 people were immune and stayed healthy. There were three people who were infected but three people who also stayed healthy. As one can tell, the disease does not do much damage in this population.

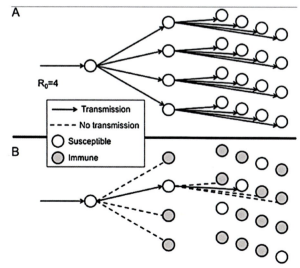

Figure 2. Diagram of herd immunity[1]

How can we achieve herd immunity? It can be achieved by vaccinating the right percentage of people in each population. Below is a chart that shows the vaccination rates necessary to achieve herd immunity:

Table 1. Herd Immunity Thresholds for some VPDs

Disease	Percentage Needed
Measles	83-94%
Mumps	75-86%
Rubella	83-85%
Diphtheria	85%
Pertussis	92-94%

% vaccination needed to achieve herd immunity

The type of disease also matters for herd immunity. One example is tetanus. As mentioned in an earlier chapter, tetanus can't be spread from person to person. The vaccination only protects oneself. For that reason, herd immunity cannot be applied to this disease. It's still important to get that vaccine so you aren't at risk. However, in terms of herd immunity, there aren't any issues. As you can see, for other diseases, herd immunity is very important. Pertussis for instance is spread through respiratory transmission. It requires a higher herd immunity threshold because it can be spread so quickly.

Let's think about "creating the herd" now. For the most part, there are many people who believe it is not their job to protect other people. In a way, empathy and compassion are very important in order for vaccines to work. What if you suddenly develop cancer? You are now an immunocompromised person. Suddenly, other people and their decisions affect your life. Except, for some people, they genuinely do not understand until it is them in that position. That's when they realize they need another person's support.

Many parents who do not support vaccines claim that it is not the job of their children to protect other children. For instance, a common slogan is "My child does not protect you". However, these parents do not realize that their decisions can negatively impact the people surrounding them. For example, there are children who have leukemia. The parents of these children have to work extra hard to find daycares and schools. They have to make sure that the children at that location are vaccinated because a common cold can cause their child to die. These parents have to work harder to protect their children and some people don't notice until it's their situation.

The parents of healthy children claim it is their right not to vaccinate. In all honesty, it's more of a privilege. In the United States, the prevalence of disease has been lowered enough that we are lucky not to worry about these diseases. Public health officials, scientists, health care workers, politicians, educators, and so many others have worked to achieve this sort of protection. Except, people just take it for granted. There are so many countries in the world right now that are trying their hardest to get as many vaccines as possible to their people. Yet, in more developed countries, there are people opting out of the opportunity to receive protection.

In a way, a healthy person can think about herd immunity as their way of helping their community. It is a social responsibility to make sure you are not harming other people. Getting a vaccine is probably one of the more simpler ways of ensuring you help your community. This chapter was purposefully titled "Create the Herd" because instead of hiding in it, we should help create it. The next time you are getting a vaccination, think about how it helps protect you but also protects other people.

> Biggest obstacle: "It's not my job to protect other peoples kids"

Conclusion

Vaccines, as you can see, are more than shots. They have so much history. There are so many misconceptions. There is so much science and research. There are so many people who create these vaccines. There is so much money involved in creating these solutions. The best part, they are very effective. Yet, there is so much controversy.

By now, you have read so much about vaccines and you may have more questions. I very clearly support vaccines. I think they have been such an asset to protecting individuals from getting diseases. I think that they are an integral part of public health.

However, there are probably some people who think I'm fairly biased. I do want to point out that as of this moment, I am an undergraduate student. Many anti-vaccine activists attack vaccine supporters by claiming that pharmaceutical companies are paying them. I, however, am writing this book to inform other college students and people of information that I think is valuable and important. I am not being paid. Someone could also make an argument that I am much too young or naïve to be considered reliable. However, considering the number of sources, the whole semester, and the thousands of dollars I am paying for my own education, I would say that the information I am presenting is reliable.

I also wanted to take a moment to make you think about pharmaceutical companies and doctors. There is a misconception that doctors and companies make more money by making people get vaccinations[1]. There are a few problems with that. Look at vaccines from a business perspective. Vaccines prevent disease. Pharmaceutical companies would want people to get sick so they buy more of their medications. Why would they create a product that would prevent sickness? If you are cynical toward pharmaceutical companies, that may have been a bad example. Apply the same concept to doctors. Doctors technically make their livelihood from their patients being sick. They need unhealthy people in order to get paid. From a business perspective, a doctor would want their patients to stay sick because more visits equal more money. However, these people are creating and endorsing a product that is very effective and protective.

I also want to take the time that vaccines are certainly not the only reason why the prevalence of disease has decreased. Sanitation and health care have certainly improved. The way many of these diseases were spread were because of poor sewage systems and poor hygiene[1]. These developments certainly played a role. However, as one can see, the graphs from the Vaccine Preventable Diseases chapter show that there were significant decreases in cases after the introduction of the vaccines.

With that being said, there is one more concept to understand when looking at scientific data. This concept is known as the illusory correlation. The illusory correlation is the idea that when two things correlate, one must cause the other. Now, that is far from the truth. Many things can correlate, but they do not show if there is causation. In order to determine if there is a link, there must be ample research and evidence. In the cases of vaccine preventable diseases, high vaccination rates definitely cause prevalence of disease to decrease significantly. However, the concept of illusory correlation is just another tool for you to keep for your future adventures.

This book has covered the basic science behind the immune system and vaccines. It went over the different types of vaccines and many of the vaccine preventable diseases. There was information on the flu and how the flu vaccine is very important in preventing pandemics. This book also covered the specifics of meningococcal meningitis. It provided extensive information regarding sexually transmitted diseases and how to avoid them. Within that chapter, there was discussion of the vaccines that can protect from two types of sexually transmitted disease.

After that, this book also tried to teach you how to navigate the online world of medical advice. I also covered information about various myths about vaccines. There was extensive information regarding the vaccines and autism myths (even though there is so much more information about it that I could tell you). This book also covered the types of ingredients that are found in vaccines along with common misconceptions. The final chapter covers how we should create the herd to help protect each other. As you can tell, that was a very large amount of information. Hopefully, you found some of it very interesting.

For all my readers who are about to go to college, get your immunization forms updated. Good luck during your first year at college! I wish you all the best in your endeavors. Have fun! Stay safe! Get new experiences! As cliché as it sounds, the college years are truly life changing and memorable.

For all my readers who may not have gone to college or are already in college or have finished college long ago, I hope this book was enlightening and maybe entertaining. All of this information is important for any human. Now that you have read and learned so much information, it's in your hands to decide:

What (should you) NOT get from college (?)

References

Introduction
1. Hamborsky, J., Kroger, A., & Wolfe, C. (. (2015). *Epidemiology and prevention of vaccine-preventable diseases* (13th ed.). United States: U.S. Dept. of Health & Human Services, Centers for Disease Control and Prevention.

Chapter 1: Background in Science
1. Hamborsky, J., Kroger, A., & Wolfe, C. (. (2015). *Epidemiology and prevention of vaccine-preventable diseases* (13th ed.). United States: U.S. Dept. of Health & Human Services, Centers for Disease Control and Prevention.
2. What are the organs of the immune system? (2013, January 14). Retrieved from https://www.ncbi.nlm.nih.gov/pubmedhealth/PMH0072579/
3. Parham, P., & Janeway, C. (2015). *The immune system.* New York, NY: Garland Science, Taylor & Francis Group.

Chapter 2: Vaccine Preventable Diseases
1. Hamborsky, J., Kroger, A., & Wolfe, C. (. (2015). *Epidemiology and prevention of vaccine-preventable diseases* (13th ed.). United States: U.S. Dept. of Health & Human Services, Centers for Disease Control and Prevention.
2. Measles. (2018, January 19). Retrieved February, 2018, from http://www.who.int/mediacentre/factsheets/fs286/en/
3. Harvard T.H. Chan School of Public Health. (2018, March 21). Mumps resurgence likely due to waning vaccine-derived immunity. *ScienceDaily*. Retrieved April 18, 2018 from www.sciencedaily.com/releases/2018/03/180321141401.htm
4. Children's Hospital. (2014, August 18). A Look at Each Vaccine: Hepatitis A Vaccine. Retrieved March, 2018, from http://www.chop.edu/centers-programs/vaccine-education-center/vaccine-details/hepatitis-a-vaccine
5. Aliferis, L. (2015, January 22). Disneyland Measles Outbreak Hits 59 Cases And Counting. Retrieved from https://www.npr.org/sections/health-shots/2015/01/22/379072061/disneyland-measles-outbreak-hits-59-cases-and-counting
6. Mina, M. J., Metcalf, C. J. E., de Swart, R. L., Osterhaus, A. D. M. E., & Grenfell, B. T. (2015). Long-term measles-induced immunomodulation increases overall childhood infectious disease mortality. *Science (New York, N.Y.), 348*(6235), 694–699. http://doi.org/10.1126/science.aaa3662
7. "Poliomyelitis." *World Health Organization*, World Health Organization, www.who.int/en/news-room/fact-sheets/detail/poliomyelitis.
8. Pertussis. (2015, September 04). Retrieved from http://www.who.int/immunization/diseases/pertussis/en/

Chapter 3: Do I Have to Get the Flu Shot?
1. Influenza (Flu). (2017, September 27). Retrieved March, 2018, from https://www.cdc.gov/flu/about/viruses/types.htm

2. Hamborsky, J., Kroger, A., & Wolfe, C. (. (2015). *Epidemiology and prevention of vaccine-preventable diseases* (13th ed.). United States: U.S. Dept. of Health & Human Services, Centers for Disease Control and Prevention.
3. Case file: The Flu Krew. (2015, December 18). Retrieved from https://www.cdc.gov/bam/diseases/immune/db/flu.html
4. Taubenberger, J. K., & Morens, D. M. (2006). 1918 Influenza: the Mother of All Pandemics. *Emerging Infectious Diseases*, *12*(1), 15–22. http://doi.org/10.3201/eid1201.050979
5. Al-Muharrmi, Z. (2010). Understanding the Influenza A H1N1 2009 Pandemic. *Sultan Qaboos University Medical Journal*, *10*(2), 187–195.
6. Influenza (Flu). (2014, July 17). Retrieved from https://www.cdc.gov/flu/about/qa/1918flupandemic.htm
7. Del Rio, C., & Guarner, J. (2010). The 2009 Influenza A (H1N1) Pandemic: What Have We Learned in the Past 6 Months. *Transactions of the American Clinical and Climatological Association*, *121*, 128–140.
8. Saunders-Hastings, P. R., & Krewski, D. (2016). Reviewing the History of Pandemic Influenza: Understanding Patterns of Emergence and Transmission. *Pathogens*, *5*(4), 66. http://doi.org/10.3390/pathogens5040066
9. Seasonal influenza reviews. (2017, December 18). Retrieved from http://www.who.int/influenza/surveillance_monitoring/updates/GIP_surveillance_summary_reviews_archives/en/ Update Images: http://www.who.int/influenza/surveillance_monitoring/updates/2018_04_16_surveillance_update_313.pdf?ua=1

Chapter 4: Meningitis
1. Hamborsky, J., Kroger, A., & Wolfe, C. (. (2015). *Epidemiology and prevention of vaccine-preventable diseases* (13th ed.). United States: U.S. Dept. of Health & Human Services, Centers for Disease Control and Prevention.
2. Herlihy, S. M., & Hagood, E. (2015). *Your Baby's Best Shot: Why Vaccines are Safe and Save Lives*. Lanham, MD: Rowman & Littlefield.Foreword Written by Dr. Paul Offit
3. Statistics and Disease Facts. (n.d.). Retrieved April, 2018, from http://www.nmaus.org/disease-prevention-information/statistics-and-disease-facts/
4. Who is at risk? (n.d.). Retrieved April, 2018, from http://www.nmaus.org/disease-prevention-information/who-is-at-risk/
5. What are the symptoms? (n.d.). Retrieved April, 2018, from http://www.nmaus.org/disease-prevention-information/what-are-the-symptoms/
6. How is it spread? (n.d.). Retrieved April, 2018, from http://www.nmaus.org/disease-prevention-information/how-is-it-spread/
7. How can it be prevented? (n.d.). Retrieved April, 2018, from http://www.nmaus.org/disease-prevention-information/how-can-it-be-prevented/
8. Serogroup B Meningococcal Disease. (n.d.). Retrieved April, 2018, from http://www.nmaus.org/disease-prevention-information/serogroup-b-meningococcal-disease/

9. Serogroup B Vaccines. (n.d.). Retrieved April, 2018, from http://www.nmaus.org/disease-prevention-information/serogroup-b-meningococcal-disease/serogroup-b-vaccines/
10. Meningitis. (2018, April 10). Retrieved April, 2018, from http://www.who.int/emergencies/diseases/meningitis/en/
11. Complications of meningitis. (n.d.). Retrieved April 17, 2018, from https://www.hse.ie/eng/health/az/m/meningitis/complications-of-meningitis.html
12. nmaus2. "The Brisons' Meningitis Story - Get Vaccinated." *YouTube*, YouTube, 15 Aug. 2015, www.youtube.com/watch?v=jjIY0XTzsn0&feature=youtu.be&ab_channel=NationalMeningitisAssociation.
13. nmaus2. "Patti Wukovits's Meningitis Story - Get Vaccinated." *YouTube*, YouTube, 10 Jan. 2015, www.youtube.com/watch?v=ASg5Pef4WuM&feature=youtu.be&ab_channel=NationalMeningitisAssociation.

Chapter 5: Let's Talk Sex

1. Chlamydia. (2017, October 04). Retrieved April 18, 2018, from https://www.cdc.gov/std/chlamydia/stdfact-chlamydia.htm
2. Get Tested | National HIV, STD, and Hepatitis Testing. (n.d.). Retrieved April, 2018, from https://gettested.cdc.gov/
3. Human Papillomavirus (HPV). (n.d.). Retrieved April, 2018, from http://www.health.gov.au/internet/main/publishing.nsf/Content/ohp-HPV.htm
4. Parenthood, P. (n.d.). Birth Control Methods & Options | Types of Birth Control. Retrieved April, 2018, from https://www.plannedparenthood.org/learn/birth-control
5. Sexually Transmitted Diseases (STDs). (2017, July 03). Retrieved from https://www.cdc.gov/std/EPT/legal/default.htm
6. Women's Health Care Physicians. (n.d.). Retrieved from https://www.acog.org/Clinical-Guidance-and-Publications/Committee-Opinions/Committee-on-Gynecologic-Practice/Expedited-Partner-Therapy-in-the-Management-of-Gonorrhea-and-Chlamydial-Infection
7. Chlamydia. (2017, October 31). Retrieved from https://www.cdc.gov/std/chlamydia/treatment.htm
8. Gonorrhea. (2017, October 04). Retrieved from https://www.cdc.gov/std/gonorrhea/stdfact-gonorrhea.htm
9. Gonorrhea. (2017, October 31). Retrieved from https://www.cdc.gov/std/gonorrhea/treatment.htm
10. 2015 Sexually Transmitted Diseases Treatment Guidelines. (2018, January 04). Retrieved from https://www.cdc.gov/std/tg2015/gonorrhea.htm
11. Genital Herpes. (2017, September 01). Retrieved from https://www.cdc.gov/std/herpes/stdfact-herpes.htm
12. General HIV Information | HIV Risk Reduction Tool | CDC. (n.d.). Retrieved from https://wwwn.cdc.gov/hivrisk/what_is/what_is_hiv.html

13. Content Source: HIV.gov Date last updated: May 15, 2017. (2017, August 31). Symptoms of HIV. Retrieved from https://www.hiv.gov/hiv-basics/overview/about-hiv-and-aids/symptoms-of-hiv
14. HIV/AIDS. (2018, March 23). Retrieved from https://www.cdc.gov/hiv/basics/prep.html
15. How do I protect myself and my partner(s) from HIV, Viral Hepatitis, and STDs? | Get Tested. (n.d.). Retrieved from https://gettested.cdc.gov/content/how-do-i-protect-myself-and-my-partners-hiv-viral-hepatitis-and-stds
16. Sexually Transmitted Diseases (STDs). (2017, June 13). Retrieved from https://www.cdc.gov/std/syphilis/stdfact-syphilis.htm
17. Viral Hepatitis. (2017, September 26). Retrieved from https://www.cdc.gov/hepatitis/populations/stds.htm
18. The National Institute for Occupational Safety and Health (NIOSH). (2010, September 28). Retrieved from https://www.cdc.gov/niosh/stopsticks/bloodborne.html
19. Human Papillomavirus (HPV). (2017, November 16). Retrieved from https://www.cdc.gov/std/hpv/stdfact-hpv.htm
20. Human Papillomavirus (HPV). (2017, July 14). Retrieved from https://www.cdc.gov/std/hpv/stdfact-hpv-and-men.htm
21. Human Papillomavirus (HPV). (n.d.). Retrieved from http://www.health.gov.au/internet/main/publishing.nsf/Content/ohp-HPV.htm
22. Jones, B. (n.d.). Australia Is Set to Become The First Country to Completely Eliminate One Type of Cancer. Retrieved from https://www.sciencealert.com/australia-eradication-human-papillomavirus-vaccine-scheme

Chapter 6: How to Process Information
1. SDSU Library and Information Access. (n.d.). Retrieved April, 2018, from https://library.sdsu.edu/reference/news/what-does-peer-review-mean
2. Bohannon, J. (2015, May 27). I Fooled Millions Into Thinking Chocolate Helps Weight Loss. Here's How. Retrieved from https://io9.gizmodo.com/i-fooled-millions-into-thinking-chocolate-helps-weight-1707251800
3. Cohen, P. (2015, May 29). How the "chocolate diet" hoax fooled millions. Retrieved from https://www.cbsnews.com/news/how-the-chocolate-diet-hoax-fooled-millions/
4. Bohannon, J., Diana, K., Homm, P., & Driehaus, A. (2015). Chocolate with high Cocoa content as a weight-loss accelerator. *INTERNATIONAL ARCHIVES OF MEDICINE,8*(55). doi:10.3823/1654
5. Children's Hospital of Philadelphia. (n.d.). About the Vaccine Education Center. Retrieved from http://www.chop.edu/centers-programs/vaccine-education-center/about
6. About National Vaccine Information Center. (n.d.). Retrieved from https://www.nvic.org/about.aspx
7. Herlihy, S. M., & Hagood, E. (2015). *Your Baby's Best Shot: Why Vaccines are Safe and Save Lives*. Lanham, MD: Rowman & Littlefield. Foreword Written by Dr. Paul Offit

8. ThinkTwice Global Vaccine Institute: Avoid Vaccine Reactions. (n.d.). Retrieved from http://thinktwice.com/
9. Stromberg, J. (2014, November 21). "Get Me Off Your Fucking Mailing List" is an actual science paper accepted by a journal. Retrieved from https://www.vox.com/2014/11/21/7259207/scientific-paper-scam
10. About the AAP. (n.d.). Retrieved from https://www.aap.org/en-us/about-the-aap/Pages/About-the-AAP.aspx
11. Centers for Disease Control and Prevention. (2017, April 26). Retrieved from https://www.cdc.gov/
12. Natural Health Information Articles and Health Newsletter by Dr. Joseph Mercola. (n.d.). Retrieved from https://www.mercola.com/

Chapter 7: Myths
1. Herlihy, S. M., & Hagood, E. (2015). *Your Baby's Best Shot: Why Vaccines are Safe and Save Lives*. Lanham, MD: Rowman & Littlefield.Foreword Written by Dr. Paul Offit
2. Fitzpatrick, M. (2006). The Cutter Incident: How America's First Polio Vaccine Led to a Growing Vaccine Crisis. *Journal of the Royal Society of Medicine*, *99*(3), 156.
3. Vaccine Safety. (2018, January 26). Retrieved from https://www.cdc.gov/vaccinesafety/concerns/multiple-vaccines-immunity.html
4. Offit, Paul A., et al. "Addressing Parents' Concerns: Do Multiple Vaccines Overwhelm or Weaken the Infant's Immune System?" *Pediatrics*, American Academy of Pediatrics, 1 Jan. 2002, pediatrics.aappublications.org/content/109/1/124.
5. Offit, P. A. (2015). *Deadly Choices: How the Anti-vaccine Movement Threatens Us All*. New york: Basic Books.

Chapter 8: Autism
1. Offit, P. A. (2010). *Autism's False Prophets: Bad Science, Risky Medicine, and the Search for a Cure*. NY: Columbia University Press.
2. Herlihy, S. M., & Hagood, E. (2015). *Your Baby's Best Shot: Why Vaccines are Safe and Save Lives*. Lanham, MD: Rowman & Littlefield.Foreword Written by Dr. Paul Offit
3. RETRACTED: Ileal-lymphoid-nodular hyperplasia, non-specific colitis, and pervasive developmental disorder in children Wakefield, AJ et al. The Lancet, Volume 351, Issue 9103 , 637 – 641
4. Autism Spectrum Disorder (ASD). (2016, April 18). Retrieved from https://www.cdc.gov/ncbddd/autism/hcp-dsm.html
5. Sharfstein JM. Vaccines and the Trump Administration. *JAMA*. 2017;317(13):1305–1306. doi:10.1001/jama.2017.2311
6. Robbins, R. (2018, April 19). Meeting with Trump emboldens anti-vaccine activists. Retrieved from https://www.statnews.com/2016/11/30/donald-trump-vaccines-policy/

7. Offit, P. A. (2015). *Deadly Choices: How the Anti-vaccine Movement Threatens Us All*. New york: Basic Books.

Chapter 9: Ingredients
1. Herlihy, S. M., & Hagood, E. (2015). *Your Baby's Best Shot: Why Vaccines are Safe and Save Lives*. Lanham, MD: Rowman & Littlefield. Foreword Written by Dr. Paul Offit
2. Children's Hospital. (2014, November 06). Vaccine Ingredients – Fetal Tissues. Retrieved from http://www.chop.edu/centers-programs/vaccine-education-center/vaccine-ingredients/fetal-tissues
3. Offit, Paul. "Vaccine Ingredients – Corn and Peanut Oils." *Children's Hospital of Philadelphia*, The Children's Hospital of Philadelphia, 27 Sept. 2016, www.chop.edu/centers-programs/vaccine-education-center/vaccine-ingredients/corn-and-peanut-oils.
4. Offit, Paul. "Vaccine Ingredients - Aluminum." *Children's Hospital of Philadelphia*, The Children's Hospital of Philadelphia, 22 Mar. 2018, www.chop.edu/centers-programs/vaccine-education-center/vaccine-ingredients/aluminum.
5. Casella, C. R., & Mitchell, T. C. (2008). Putting endotoxin to work for us: monophosphoryl lipid A as a safe and effective vaccine adjuvant. *Cellular and Molecular Life Sciences : CMLS*, 65(20), 3231–3240. http://doi.org/10.1007/s00018-008-8228-6
6. Jefferson, T., Rudin, M., & Pietrantonj, C. D. (2004). Adverse events after immunisation with aluminum-containing DTP vaccines: Systematic review of the evidence. *The Lancet Infectious Diseases,4*(2), 84-90. doi:10.1016/s1473-3099(04)00927-2
7. Children's Hospital. (2014, November 06). Vaccine Ingredients – Formaldehyde. Retrieved from http://www.chop.edu/centers-programs/vaccine-education-center/vaccine-ingredients/formaldehyde
8. Techniques Lab A. (n.d.). Retrieved from http://www.accessexcellence.org/AE/AEPC/geneconn/smallvol.html
9. Enfamil Infant Formula, Powder, 12.5 oz Can (Case of 6). (2018, April 27). Retrieved from https://www.enfamil.com/products/enfamil-infant/12-5-oz-powder-can-case-6?gclid=EAIaIQobChMIpZOl-YWx2gIVmUwNCh12Mw5TEAYYAiABEgL2PfD_BwE
10. DORITOS® Nacho Cheese Flavored Tortilla Chips. (n.d.). Retrieved from https://www.fritolay.com/snacks/product-page/doritos/doritos-nacho-cheese-flavored-tortilla-chips
11. Ingredients of All-Natural Blueberries. (2014, February 24). Retrieved from https://jameskennedymonash.wordpress.com/2013/12/20/ingredients-of-all-natural-blueberries/

Chapter 10: Create the Herd
1. Paul Fine, Ken Eames, David L. Heymann; "Herd Immunity": A Rough Guide, *Clinical Infectious Diseases*, Volume 52, Issue 7, 1 April 2011, Pages 911–916, https://doi.org/10.1093/cid/cir007
2. Helft, Emily Willingham and Laura. "What Is Herd Immunity?" *PBS*, Public Broadcasting Service, 5 Sept. 2014, www.pbs.org/wgbh/nova/body/herd-immunity.html.
3. Harris, R., Popovich, N., Powell, K., & Team, G. U. (n.d.). Watch how the measles outbreak spreads when kids get vaccinated – and when they don't. Retrieved from https://www.theguardian.com/society/ng-interactive/2015/feb/05/-sp-watch-how-measles-outbreak-spreads-when-kids-get-vaccinated

Conclusion
1. Herlihy, S. M., & Hagood, E. (2015). *Your Baby's Best Shot: Why Vaccines are Safe and Save Lives*. Lanham, MD: Rowman & Littlefield.Foreword Written by Dr. Paul Offit

Made in the USA
Middletown, DE
28 August 2019